S0-AFK-224

TABLE OF CONTENTS

PREFACE

You're probably wondering why you have to read yet another book about diabetes. As if having the disease isn't bad enough! But take it from us, it's better to spend the time learning about diabetes than to take stupid risks. You might also be wondering who we are, anyway, talking about something you already know plenty about. Well, we're a couple of people who have diabetes ourselves and teach people how to live with it. Jean is a nurse who now has three young adult children and who herself developed diabetes while in college. Sue is a dietitian and has one child of her own—a Labrador retriever. She diagnosed her own diabetes when she was 14. We met several years ago and soon became friends.

Diabetes is a serious condition, and yet, we've found that it doesn't have to be a big drag. We figure, make the best of what you've been given and get on with things. What's the point of complaining about something you can't change? One of the best ways we've handled the trials of diabetes is to keep our sense of humor. We might give diabetes some grief, but if Steve Martin can make parenthood funny, we figure diabetes is fair game. As Plato once said, "Even the gods love jokes!"

Being a teen is hard enough. You have to worry about dating, your family, drugs and alcohol, friendships, and changes in your body. Who needs the added frustration of diabetes? We hope this book will give you some help so that even when diabetes gets you down, getting back up is no big deal.

Introduction

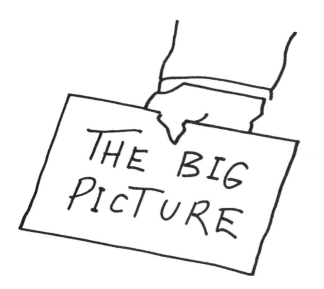

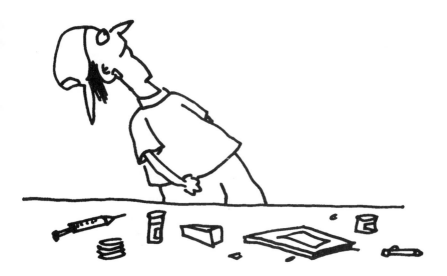

In Control

So you have diabetes. Not the best of news, but it's better than being stuck in a desert with no water and a lame camel. It might be worse than three term papers all due on the same afternoon or having to baby-sit your annoying cousins, but that's a close call.

The good news is that diabetes can be managed. Putting it into the big picture is important, though. You should ask yourself how diabetes fits into your life. We're old pros at juggling diabetes and busy schedules. But we're not teens, and times have changed. We remember when movies were 50 cents and we had to walk ten miles through waist-high snow just to get to the bus stop . . . (on second thought, we'll leave that story for your grandparents).

Living with diabetes as a teen is hardly a walk in the park. Nobody understands that better than people who have gone through the same thing and are still dealing with diabetes. Sometimes (when you're in an ugly mood), don't you just wish you could switch places with someone else so they could appreciate what you're going through? We would love to exchange a day (or more) of freedom from diabetes with anyone who thinks they can tell us how we should live with this disease. (In fact, getting friends and relatives to try it out by following a meal plan, testing blood and urine, and taking injections of saline can be very interesting.)

There are a lot of things that can make diabetes more of a pain in the neck than it already is (if that's possible): well–meaning relatives who just don't seem to have a clue, insensitive friends and kids at school, overprotective parents, the unpredictability of the big "D" itself, the hormone horrors that send your blood sugar level reeling, doing all sorts of wonderful tasks that no one else needs to worry about, and the ever-present questions about the future.

We've heard people wail, "What did I ever do to deserve diabetes?" Sure, having diabetes is tough and it's not going away. But if you haven't already learned that life isn't always fair, now is as good a time as any. You have to play the hand you're dealt, take your injections, and move on. No one "deserves" any disease. There was nothing you could have done to prevent yourself from getting it.

So the question now is, "What are you going to do about it?" You can spend a lot of time being mopey and ticked off—*that's* a good use of your energy. Or there's always the option of fitting it into your life and getting on with it. It's like being stuck with the body you've got when you know in your heart you were meant to have the body of Cindy Crawford or Arnold Schwarzenegger. The fact remains that you still have to live with your skinny bird's legs or oversized middle. Unfortunately, diabetes also comes with the package.

Diabetes is kind of like a little brother. Usually he's a big pain, but every once in a while he actually does something nice, making your life just a little bit better. Diabetes is your unchosen partner in life, and while it may seem to be more like a jail sentence, it can also teach you a lot about yourself and other people—if you let it.

Speaking Frankly ♦ ♦ ♦

There are a couple of things we want to tell you about how we deal with diabetes. You'll probably notice this in the way we write and speak.

Diabetic—We prefer not to be "diabetic," but to be people with diabetes. Just because we have diabetes doesn't mean we don't exist as people. It might sound picky, but you don't hear of heart–attackics or hemorrhoidics too often now, do you? You may have heard people use diabetic to describe different food types such as diabetic cake or diabetic ice cream. A cake with diabetes? Sure, and my dog plays lead guitar with Aerosmith.

Normal–Many people continue to use the words "diabetic" and "normal" to describe research groups, blood glucose levels, and people who don't have diabetes. But we know plenty of people without diabetes who don't exactly fit into the "normal" category. If you think about it, normal is just a relative concept anyway.

Good, not good, or bad–Some people say blood sugar levels are "good, not good, or bad." This is only a value judgment! We want our blood sugar levels to be in range, within goal ranges, in target range, or to be high or low, not good or bad. Too many people start to think if their blood sugar levels are not "good," they must be "bad." Your blood sugar is neither good nor bad. It may be high or low, and you may know why or have no clue. Either way, don't blame yourself or let other people bug you about something you had no control over or a decision you did or didn't make.

Target range–When we refer to your target range, we mean the goal blood sugar levels that you and your doctor have agreed upon. If you don't have a target range to shoot for, you might want to have a little chat with your doctor or diabetes treatment team.

Insulin shock or reaction–Here's where our personal pet peeves come in. Jean particularly objects to the word "reaction" and Sue dislikes "shock" (both meaning low blood sugar). These are old-fashioned and imprecise terms describing low blood sugar or hypoglycemia. Low blood sugar is not a true "shock" and people confuse "reaction" with allergic reactions to drugs. Neither one is correct—just another example of how the English language is going right down the tubes. (A little melodrama never hurt anyone.)

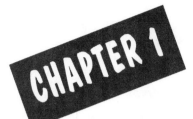

CHAPTER 1

YOU:
LEADING THE WAY

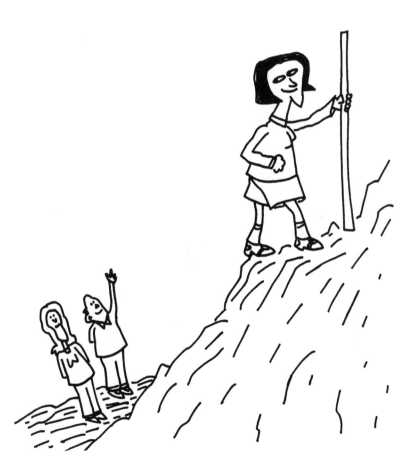

GETTING A GRIP!

When you first got diabetes, you may or may not have counted on your parents to help you with all the things you needed to do to take care of yourself. Teens usually handle diabetes better when their parents have some input, but the question is when does their control become too much? One way of solving this is to take charge of your blood testing and injections yourself, let your mom fix the healthy meals, and ask your dad to order supplies and help with insulin changes. Or you could take care of most of it yourself and ask your parents for help when a problem comes up.

Let's back up and talk about the good old days, when you were younger and your parents did almost everything for you (assuming you've had diabetes for a while). You felt safe and protected knowing they would take care of you, and they felt they had some control over the way your diabetes was managed. At that point, your diabetes was probably more easily controlled.

However, all this changes when you go through that wonderful stage: puberty. You've probably heard plenty of jokes about the various changes your body goes through and experienced a lot of it first-hand. You may feel moodier than usual and your parents may start to really get on your nerves. ("A 10:30 curfew? What am I? Four years old?") You might also start to resent all the things they try to do for you, instead of letting you do them yourself. The biggest culprits for this confusion are the different hormones* your body is producing.

---

*A hormone, basically, is a chemical made in one part of your body that travels in the bloodstream and affects other parts of the body. Examples of hormones are: growth hormones (help you grow), thyroid hormones (affect your metabolism), sex hormones (help you develop into a man or woman), and adrenaline or epinephrine (made under stress).

While you may have covered this territory in school, what you won't hear about is how these hormones affect your diabetes. They actually cause the insulin you take to work less effectively, and your blood sugar level can go up.

So now what? On one hand, we have your parents, who love you and feel shut out when you suddenly decide to become independent. On the other hand, we have you, a growing teenager who wants to be your own person. Sometimes parents (and even you, yourself) don't know how to react to this. They might just let you do your own thing and then worry a lot. Or they might try to keep some control over your diabetes and intrude on your space.

So here you are, trying to be independent while your blood sugar levels become higher because of the hormones and people start blaming you for not taking care of yourself. Frank was in a similar predicament:

Frank was 13 years old, having had diabetes since he was five. Over the years, his blood sugar level had been in and out of his target range, but mostly in. He always tested his blood and urine, always took his insulin, and only sometimes went off his meal plan. He frequently talked to his mother about his insulin dose, and she would make sure he had the right amount drawn up in the syringe.

When Frank entered the wonderful world of teenhood, he started giving his own shots and didn't bother talking to his mom anymore about doses. He was proud that he was comfortable and able to make the adjustment and give the insulin himself. In fact, it was much easier this way, since his mom worked and wasn't always around.

In Control

At the same time, Frank noticed that his voice was changing, his shoes were almost always too small, and suddenly he wasn't so short anymore. He also noticed that his stomach was demanding more and more food—especially during lunch and after school. Even though he tried to limit the food he ate at lunch, it was hard because he was sure the growling would disrupt his class (he was always thinking of other people). Some of the time he stuck to his meal plan, but usually he couldn't resist having desserts and snacks with his friends. Not surprisingly, Frank's blood sugar level kept rising. It seemed like the harder he tried to keep it under control, the more his blood sugar levels bounced up and down.

When his mom saw Frank's numbers in his meter's memory, it wasn't a pretty sight. She told him she had heard (from anonymous sources, of course) that he had been eating sweets. So he decided to quit doing the readings so she wouldn't know what they were—not one of his better ideas. Without the readings, Frank couldn't adjust his insulin and his blood sugar levels remained high. His mom then got upset (had a cow) and decided that if he wasn't going to take care of himself, she was going to take away his privileges.

Finally, Frank, his parents, and his treatment team sat down to talk about what was going on. His doctor explained that during rapid growth, Frank needed more food and more insulin. In time, Frank began to understand where his parents were coming from. They were worried about his future and felt like they were losing control. In fact, Frank admitted that he wasn't quite as comfortable in the role of captain as he thought he would be. Together, they worked out a plan:

- Frank would work at doing more blood sugar tests and would write them down. (This would get his parents off his back and show them he was doing the tests.)

- Frank would show his numbers to his parents once or twice a week. His mom also promised not to freak out at the numbers, even if they were high.

- Frank and/or his mom would call the diabetes educator or Frank's doctor once a week for guidance, and they would all let each other know what the new plan was. (Calling the educator helps cut down on arguing over decisions about food and insulin between Frank and his parents.)

- Frank's mom and dad would occasionally ask if he was doing OK and if they could help out. Frank promised (this was the tough part) to tell them where he was having a hard time, such as at lunch in school. They all agreed to talk about it to work out a solution.

Frank needed to tell his parents what was going on and show them that he was taking responsibility. His parents relaxed a little, knowing that Frank was trying and that they weren't being left out if he had a problem.

This story has a happy ending, but this isn't always the case (big surprise). You may not have an educator working with you, and you or your parents may not be able to agree on anything. What do you do then? You may need to be even more creative in finding a supportive person who can help pull everyone together. This can be a social worker, clergyman, counselor, or your doctor.

> **Bottom Line:** Everyone is different—with cooperation and patience, things usually work out for the best.

YOUR OUTLOOK

"It's not so much what happens to us in life that matters, but the outlook we take toward what happens."

—Charles Woodson

Years ago when Jean was diagnosed with diabetes, she kept a poster that said, "When life hands out lemons, make lemonade." There was a rainbow in the picture and lots of glasses of lemonade. She remembers thinking, "Sure, and I'll bet that lemonade has sugar in it . . . ." The irony of it all. She believes in the philosophy that you should expect the worst but hope for the best. It might sound a little pessimistic, but it's really just realistic. The idea is the old Boy Scout motto: "Be Prepared." It's a matter of thinking ahead and planning for roadblocks before they come up.

Now, we're not singing diabetes' praises. Hardly! But there have been the occasional bonuses that have influenced who we are and how we live our lives. "Oh, no," you might be thinking. "Not the old 'Every cloud has a silver lining' routine."

Well, diabetes doesn't really make your life more wonderful, and you DO need to look pretty hard for the positive aspects of the disease. But just as with other misfortunes, if you look hard enough you can usually find something good that comes out of it. There's an old Chinese proverb that goes something like, "Disaster breeds opportunity." There may be a few things you can think of that have been pluses for you. Write them down so you can dredge them up and dust them off when you're having a down day.

Here are some positive comments we've heard from teens:

—*"Well, diabetes has made me learn to be disciplined . . . which I never was before. Actually, it's made me more disciplined with sports and school work."*

—*"I think I have more respect for my body than other kids my age. I have a better understanding that health is important. I don't use tobacco or drink, and I don't eat a lot of high fat foods. I also get more exercise, and I think these patterns will make me healthier in the future. In fact, sometimes I feel healthier than my friends."*

—*"My family eats better now. Before my diabetes, my dad had high blood pressure and my mom was overweight. Since they've been eating healthier, they're both doing better."*

—*"Watching what I eat and exercising has helped me keep a healthy weight. A lot of my friends have gained weight, and they don't know what foods to avoid to not gain weight."*

—*"I think I have more understanding and acceptance of other people. I know what it's like to feel different."*

Sometimes those of us with diabetes work harder at something just to show others we won't let it keep us down. We both feel that diabetes has enriched our lives in some ways. Having had an uncertain illness for a long time has helped us both appreciate each moment along the way. That has been a gift.

> **Bottom Line: Focus on the positive.**

WHEN DIABETES MESSES UP YOUR LIFE . . .

Diabetes isn't ALWAYS to blame when something upsetting happens. (We know, it often feels that way.) And things that upset you can certainly mess up your diabetes.

We've heard all kinds of horror stories:

- Nancy had ketones and threw up on prom night.
- Eric had low blood sugar during finals.
- John's football coaches benched him because they were afraid he'd have low blood sugar.
- Jennifer learned that her dream guy, Jack, wouldn't ask her out because he thought he could catch diabetes!

Sometimes everything seems to get screwed up—and you just have to deal with it. On the other hand, many times there are steps you can take to make things better.

Jean's friend, Lynn, is an avid biker who also has diabetes. Lynn would go on long biking trips with her friends. She became frustrated as diabetes messed up not only her own trips, but everyone else's plans as well. Lynn didn't usually test her blood before she went, because she was always in a hurry. She never ate much either, because her friends didn't eat a lot on the trips. As a result, sometimes she'd be biking, feel low, and have to make the whole group wait while she treated herself. She was embarrassed and sometimes her friends complained about having to stop. If Lynn was biking and felt really tired, she might eat sweets thinking she was low. (She found out later that her blood sugar wasn't low, it was actually high.) Sometimes she'd get "super thirsty" and would need to stop to find a restroom or drinking fountain.

Lynn finally got fed up with this routine and feeling sad that she was annoying her friends, thought about quitting biking. But she enjoyed it and decided to try to overcome her diabetes obstacles. "Taking care of my diabetes is like walking on stepping stones. If I take care of it each step along the way, I can go wherever I want," Lynn commented.

She now tests her blood before she starts biking, adjusts her insulin, and eats before leaving. She usually tests when the others take a break and adjusts her diet. "Sometimes I still get low, but much less often than before. And my friends aren't so worried about me. Actually they seem happy that I'm taking care of myself, and I feel better too," Lynn added. Of course, it does take extra time to do these things, but in the end it saves a lot of aggravation.

Our friend Richard has two **"Rules to Live By:"**

1. *Make diabetes as small a part of your life as possible.* Ask yourself what this really means to you. If you push your diabetes away, you may end up feeling guilt, regret, anger, and lots of high and low blood sugar. Diabetes is portable—you can run but you can't hide. So you need to fit it in without a lot of moaning and groaning.

2. *You can do almost anything you want with diabetes as long as you figure out where you have to give.* In other words, there's a diabetes give and take. In order to accomplish something, you may need to give something up. You know, the yin for the yang! Figure out the necessary adjustments you can handle to fit diabetes into your life.

In Control

Carol wrote, *"I remember in my first year with diabetes, I had a big physics test. I was nervous and cramming to study. Instead of lunch, I decided to keep on studying. As a result, my blood sugar dropped during the test and I had to leave the room. After class I went to explain to my teacher what had happened. He gave me an F on my test and said I deserved it because I should have known not to skip a meal. He was right, and I've never done it again!"* The message: Don't forget the little steps.

Lydia, on the other hand, was often tired, sick to her stomach, and forced to miss school. She was referred to a counselor for help, who found out that Lydia's favorite pastime was going to the mall with her friends, which she did pretty much every day. Lydia liked to eat there but didn't feel like taking her insulin while she was with her friends. When she got home, she figured it was too late to take it, so she just skipped her second shot and then missed school the next day because she was nauseated and had high blood sugar.

After a few counseling sessions, Lydia decided that it wouldn't be such a big deal for her to take a pre–filled syringe to the mall. It would only take a few seconds to give it in a restroom, and she figured that if her friends couldn't handle it, they weren't the best friends to have anyway. This was the compromise that allowed Lydia to do what she wanted—without messing up her life.

So let's go back to the "horror" stories we talked about on page 8. Maybe a lot of grief could have been avoided if:

- Nancy hadn't gotten so caught up in prom and graduation activities that she forgot to take her insulin.

- Eric had tested his blood and made sure he had eaten his snack before his exam.

- John had talked to his football coach and explained diabetes, or had his parents or diabetes educator give the coach information. John could also show his coach that he was taking care of himself by checking his blood sugar and keeping glucose tablets on hand.

- Jennifer had taken the chance to spend some time explaining diabetes to her close friends rather than avoiding the topic.

Richard (of "Richard's Rules") has also identified a condition that he calls your "sticking point." It's kind of like hitting an ungreased part of a greased slide. You're trying to move forward, but there's something you have to get through to move on. When you stick, it slows you down. You probably already know the things that hold you back.

The process of trying to find out what your sticking point is and how to move around it is a little trick called problem solving. It's the process of deciding where you stick, why you got stuck, how to get yourself moving, and how to prevent yourself from getting stuck the next time.

> **Bottom Line:** Know your sticking points and unglue yourself.

Diabetes (that little pest) also got in Mark's way when he wanted to go skydiving. His mom, worrying that his diabetes might cause him problems, called Mark's doctor and nurse and strongly asked that they forbid him to jump due to his diabetes. The medical staff, however, felt that as long as he checked his blood sugar levels, there was no diabetes-related reason he couldn't jump. On the big day, it was the skydiving crew that cancelled the jump when they learned of Mark's diabetes. (They were afraid of being sued!) Once again, one of life's unfair moments came shining through.

Yes, diabetes can mess you up. But we don't know anyone who doesn't have some problem, and the best advice we can give is to not dwell on it, find the humor in it if you can, and GET ON with things. Easier said than done, right? Try to accept what can't be changed and take charge of the rest.

> **Bottom Line:** Diabetes can mess things up for you, but if you take the steps to take care of yourself, you can avoid a lot of grief!!

REAL NUMBERS FOR REAL TEENS

"My numbers? I forgot them—they're at home on the refrigerator."

"My dog ate them."

"I lost my paper . . . ."

"They're written down in my notebook—I left it at school."

"Some of the numbers that are on my page aren't in the memory; they're from my other meter. No, I didn't bring it."

"I thought you wanted my blood to always be between 80 and 120 (4.4 and 6.6 millimols per liter * [mmol/L])!"

"Does it say 321 (17.8 mmol/L) in the memory? I must have gotten it backwards when I wrote down 123 (6.8)!"

**Outside the U.S., blood glucose is often measured in millimols per liter (mmol/L). To convert a test result in milligrams per deciliter (mg/dL) into mmol/L, simply divide the number by 18. For instance, 140 mg/dL divided by 18 equals 7.7 mmol/L.*

As diabetes educators, there isn't a whole lot you can get past us. We know how many people write down incorrect numbers in their daily records. (Sue refers to this as "delusional glucose levels.") If you've ever done this, you're not alone!

The question is why people do it and what can be done to help them stop? Now, with meters that have a memory, it's a little bit harder to get away with writing down bogus numbers. Jean has seen teens:

- sit in the waiting room before their doctor's appointment, making up numbers and writing them down.

- ask friends to test blood on their meter to get some low readings recorded.*

- play with fingernail polish, jelly, and sugar water to make up readings rather than test real blood.

- write down 148 when blood is really 348, 114 for 214, or 102 for 201 (In millimols per liter, write down 8.2 when blood is really 10.2.)

- wonder how numbers miraculously appear in the record book, but aren't in the memory of their only meter.

What's going on here? Your parents, doctors, educators, and others have expectations of you and how you should take care of yourself. You, on the other hand, find it hard to do all this stuff, keeping diabetes management a priority and everything. When you have homework, chores, school activities, dates, basketball practice, parties, and maybe a job, it's pretty hard to keep everything straight— even if you want to. Sometimes, one of the following happens:

*Follow the manufacturer's instructions for cleaning and safety when sharing the use of your meter and finger pricking device. Never share "end–caps" on the finger pricking devices unless properly cleaned in bleach solution.

– You don't do the testing but feel like you should have something written down for your appointment. After all, it's expected and the pressure will be on.

– You did the testing but forgot or didn't take time to write it down.

– You didn't want your parents to freak out at the numbers.

– You figured there was no point in testing since you'd been totally off your meal plan, feeling high, and could guess what your blood sugar was.

– You felt guilty because you knew you did something to cause a high number and didn't want your parents to give you the third degree.

Don't kid yourself! Sue and Jean have been on both sides of this fence. You definitely aren't kidding your doctor (who knows that when your HbA$_1$C* is 11 and your numbers are all 70 to 150 [3.9 to 8.3 mmol/L], something is wrong). Whose numbers are they, anyway? Rather than hide them because they aren't what you or someone else thinks they should be, take the steering wheel, the driver's seat, or the upper hand to make them that way.

> **Bottom Line: Act, don't react! Work to make things the way you want them to be! What you don't know can hurt you!**

You're not perfect (at least, not always, right?) and we know this stuff can be hard. But nobody is perfect, and neither Sue nor Jean (mighty experts on high) has met a person who copes perfectly with their diabetes management. Sometimes no matter how hard you try or how logical your decisions are, blood test results don't

*A glycosylated hemoglobin (HbA$_1$C or HbA$_1$) test measures your average blood sugar level over the past two months.

end up where you want them to be. There are just too many things that can change from one day to the next. This includes how well your insulin is absorbed, your activity level, the foods you eat and when you eat them, and how much stress you might be under. Some people, however, do seem to do better than others.

Why is that, you ask? (All right, so you didn't ask, but we're going to tell you anyway.)

1. Some people are just plain LUCKY! (Not many qualify in this category.)

2. Some people keep on trying. They don't have an "all or nothing" approach. They keep plugging away.

3. Other people have studied their illness and know it and their body *so* well that they make excellent decisions.

4. A few people have relatively stress-free lives and stick to a schedule.

Many of us don't fall into any of these categories. Jean thinks she's a No.2 (takes a lickin' and keeps on tickin'). Sue, on the other hand, thinks she's a No.4. What category do you fit into? Or maybe you don't fit into one—yet!

All stable relationships are built on a couple of simple principles: Honesty and Integrity (the "HI" principle). Being honest and up front about your blood sugar records and what's happening in your life really helps your doctor and nurses find the best answers for you.

Integrity boils down to taking care of your body because YOU want to. You're good enough, you're smart enough, and gosh darn it, you're worth it! If you think about it, the way you act usually reflects how you feel about yourself. One guy we met seemed addicted to fast food. He hadn't bothered to ask himself why he was always pigging out, but he came to realize that it might have reflected his low self-esteem. By consciously making healthier food choices, he began to feel better about himself and more in control. In turn, he lost weight, felt better physically, and girls started paying attention.

By making up information, you're only hurting yourself. We all know that guilty feeling of going to the dentist without having flossed or going to a music lesson when you've barely practiced. It's the same thing. However, your doctor or educator will most likely want to help you with the hurdles. When you and your doctor have the benefit of real information, it will be easier to keep your blood sugar levels in range. It won't be easy, but you might find that your parents', doctor's, or treatment team's concerns are actually less of a burden than your own conscience.

If you're doing something you know you shouldn't or not doing something you know you should, it might be hard to ease your guilty conscience. Maybe someone on your health care team can help you work it out.They may not congratulate you, but they will respect you for having the guts to be honest and they'll be willing to work together. Try to find a someone you trust and with whom you can talk openly.

WHEN DIABETES ISN'T YOUR TOP PRIORITY

As a student, you're probably sort of busy. (Understatement, you say?) Not all activities and goals were invented to coexist harmoniously with diabetes. Keith wrote, "I learned a long time ago that my life shouldn't revolve around my diabetes, but that the care of my diabetes should be adjusted around my life and the many activities I have chosen. I think having a positive health attitude is a great way to confront diabetes."

When your tennis or hockey team has just made the championships, when you have a crucial final test in calculus, when you have band practice after school and homework until midnight, or when you're the lead in "Grease," it's hard to make diabetes a priority in your life.

If you don't take care of your diabetes, though, it can really get the better of you. How embarrassing to have low blood sugar in the middle of the class play and forget your lines! Better to have tested and eaten beforehand.

There will be times in your life when you and your diabetes team will have to settle for less than the tightest control. It takes a lot of energy to stay on top of diabetes every minute of every day, and when you're busy or have other priorities, that energy goes in another direction.

What do you do? When you discover yourself having trouble finding the time and energy to care for your diabetes, you have to decide for yourself what is the least you can do and still keep blood sugar levels in the best possible control. Some people may have to work harder at it than others. For example, Mike was playing championship soccer at his high school, which required long daily practices and weekend trips. He was tempted not to do blood testing or adjusting, because he rationalized that he was exercising every day and just didn't have time for it. However, he also knew that last year when he felt low, his coach pulled him out of the game and wouldn't let him finish. The season before that, when his blood sugar levels were very high, he couldn't perform well because he was tired. He decided that testing before, during, and after practice was the best thing he could do to keep up his performance.

GUIDELINES FOR KEEPING DIABETES CONTROL REASONABLE IN TIMES OF STRESS:

- Always take your insulin.

- Try to follow your usual meal times and amounts.

- Test blood sugar and urine for ketones whenever you don't feel well.

- Test blood often for special events such as an exam, performance, athletic activity, or prom.

You may need to lower your standards for times when other things in your life are overwhelming you. You probably won't have the control you're aiming for, but you should get through the tough spots without too much trouble.

Bottom Line: Create a process that prevents problems.

CHAPTER 2

REAL FOOD FOR REAL TEENS

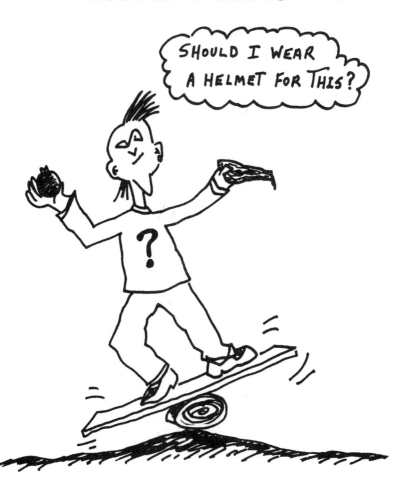

Food is a sacred subject for many of us. Questions about it might just prompt you to tell the dietitian or doctor what you believe they want to hear, instead of what they should know—what you really eat. (We can memorize what we're supposed to do. It's actually carrying it out that's the hard part!)

Wouldn't it be great if you could have your sweet tooth (and fat tooth) removed at the diagnosis of diabetes? It could solve a lot of the dilemmas you face when deciding what to eat or drink and how much. Nevertheless, those cravings for chocolate or burgers are real. So are the decisions you make and the results you get.

Some people tend to view foods on a moral scale and label them good or bad based on their nutritional content. But try exchanging the words "moral" or "immoral" for the words "good" or "bad." It's ridiculous to call a cheeseburger immoral. You don't judge people by the way they dress or the music they like, do you? You need to know what's inside them. In the same way, foods can't be completely judged on nutritional content; they also provide color, texture, contrast, taste, and fullness. They also quench your thirst.

So, describing foods as good or bad doesn't help you decide if they meet your needs. In other words, all foods have value. It just depends on how they fit into your daily schedule (and everyone's day is different). A more sensible approach is to group foods by how they fit each person as an individual and into the whole day's nutrition.

For example, a granola bar might not be such a smart choice for a 15-year-old girl trying to lose weight, but it could be just the thing for a lean 17-year-old male cross-country runner. It all depends on your body's needs.

> Bottom Line: All foods have value; view your diet in the context of a whole day or week rather than judging each food as you eat it.

People with diabetes often have to deal with busybodies who think THEY know what you should and shouldn't be eating. Do your friends ever jump down your throat just as you're biting into a Snickers? Do people get upset with you when you're eating something sweet, even though it might be because you feel low or are going to exercise, because you've planned to eat a special food, or because you've made a decision to just eat something anyway? What do you do?

Sue was invited to lunch a few years ago by a nurse she worked with. They decided to eat in the cafeteria, where the choices included the special (meatloaf, mashed potatoes, and peas) and the alternative (tuna noodle casserole). Sue thinks meatloaf is disgusting, so she opted for the tuna noodle casserole, which the cafeteria happened to make pretty well. After sitting down, the nurse started to grill Sue about why she picked the tuna casserole, since it was probably high in fat and difficult to calculate the exchanges on. After a rather tense lunch, she told the nurse that she felt awkward eating with someone who made her feel like she had to justify what she chose to eat. After all, who was the dietitian here? And more importantly, the one with the diabetes? Sue took the opportunity to teach her about current thinking on food and diabetes care.

Our friend Keith, a pharmacy professor at Washington State University and a Certified Diabetes Educator, was diagnosed with diabetes when he was 8 years old. He told us this story:

"It was probably one of the best things that ever happened to me in terms of caring for my diabetes. I was at the sensitive age when I wasn't sure I wanted a lot of people to know about my diabetes, and I especially wanted to take charge of it myself and not have someone looking over my shoulder all the time. My mother and I went downtown to Christmas shop and the local Kress store had a turkey dinner special. As we sat down to eat, my mother loudly announced to the waitress that her son had diabetes and that she would be very pleased if they would put less gravy on the potatoes and be sure to leave off any cranberry sauce. I remember looking around and it seemed like several thousand people were all staring at me and a couple of people actually moved away out of fear that they might develop diabetes. After eating, my mother and I left the store and were waiting to cross the street when I turned to her and told her that I never wanted her to ever embarrass me again about my diabetes. I was smart enough to scrape the gravy off my potatoes, not eat the cranberry sauce, and only eat a portion of the food, and I didn't need her to announce all of this to the world and embarrass me. Her response was that since I had such a big mouth and seemed to know it all, she would back out of any involvement in what I ate and let me take care of it myself. Surprisingly, she did! That was 43 years ago, and again, it was one of the best things that ever happened to me."

In the past, it was thought that teens who were independent were more successful. Now researchers have shown that most teens have lower blood sugar levels when parents stay involved with diabetes care. Most people seem to need the support and friendly interest of a family member. The trick is to find the right balance for you.

You should feel like you're in control of your own life, but know your parents are there to help. After all, no one is an island.

Another approach is to invite the "accuser" to join you. For example, Carrie had a friend who asked her why she was having a snack one day, believing that "snack" was a dirty word and people with diabetes shouldn't indulge in such things. Instead of justifying why she was eating it, Carrie said, "Yes, I'm having a snack right now, would you like to join me?"

Guilt is neither a pleasant nor helpful emotion. In fact, it's a lot like extra baggage, it only slows you down. While guilt is often laid at your feet by others, it doesn't mean you have to pick it up. It only becomes a problem for you if you accept it! You can always say to yourself: "I should have done this or I shouldn't have done that." Guilt happens when you dwell on these things. Don't "should" on yourself!

> **Bottom Line:** Do whatever works best for you and your blood sugar control and don't apologize for it!

How does all this help you make decisions about things like fast foods and sweets? Maybe we're picky, but descriptions like "fast food" and "junk food" don't seem right, either. A fast food to us is a microwavable dinner (and most of them are quite healthy these days). After all, these only take a few minutes at home, whereas a burger drive–thru can still waste a good 20 minutes of your time as you sit in line. And there are no "junk foods," just "junk diets." (Look at the forest, not the trees.) Also, many "sweets" tend to contain more fat by weight. Check out the first ingredient in most cookie, cake, and pastry desserts; it's usually butter, margarine, or lard. "Sweets" should be called something like "sweetened fat"—not too appetizing. However, all foods can have their place in the total diet, including fast foods, sweets, and junk foods.

The more important issue is how different foods affect your blood sugar levels, keeping in mind that your own body might not respond the same way as the next person's. For example, Sue's business partner, Sallie, can't even eat a small piece of pizza without her blood sugar skyrocketing. But with insulin coverage, Sue can eat three or four pieces and keep her blood sugar within range.

This is the beauty of blood sugar testing. With testing, you can get to know yourself on a level you never thought possible! And you'll find out specifically which foods you can eat more or less of, depending on your body chemistry. Sue has found that her blood sugar levels will be closer to range, or even lower, if she chooses fish instead of red meat. Also, if she substitutes an item that many people consider sweet (like an Archway cookie) in place of other carbohydrates in her diet (rice, potatoes, or noodles), there's not a huge difference in her blood sugar reading as long as the total carbohydrate intake is still the same.

Jean has found that a large vanilla Dairy Queen cone will raise her blood sugar to over 350 (19.4 mmol/L) unless she adjusts by taking eight units of Regular insulin (we'd say that's worth it!). However, try this only after discussing it with your health professionals. They have a lot of experience doing this and can help you make better judgements about your food adjustments right from the start.

For Laurie, Dairy Queen just wasn't an option. *"When I was young, my mom was very strict about what I ate. Ice cream was a big treat for me considering I was only allowed to have it once in a million years. One night after a softball game, my mom finally gave in and let me get an ice cream cone. While I was eating it, I dropped it! I was so mad at myself that I picked it up and tried to wash the ice cream off, but, of course, it didn't work.*" Now we know that testing before and after games and perhaps a small amount of insulin to cover them can let Laurie have ice cream cones without her blood sugar levels jumping up too much.

VEGETARIANISM

Vegetarianism fits into the new *Dietary Guidelines for Americans,* which promotes a diet higher in carbohydrate foods (like grains, fruits, and vegetables) and lower in animal products (dairy and meats). Studies in several countries and the United States show that people who are semi–vegetarians or vegetarians are generally healthier. (See the Food Guide Pyramid graphic on page 33). The new food guide is recommended for all Americans, but also follows what the American Diabetes Association recommends for healthy eating. So the diet that's right for you is perfect for the rest of your family, too!

Vegetarians get more than enough protein from the dairy products and eggs they might eat along with grains (an average starch exchange or serving contains about three grams of protein, which is the same as in 1/2 ounce of meat). Many people learn to work with the Food Guide Pyramid by thinking of meat as a side dish or condiment rather than the main part of the meal. Thomas Jefferson (an avid vegetable gardener and vegetarian), said nearly 100 years ago: "The flesh should be considered a condiment only." Now there's a man ahead of his time!

Types Of Vegetarians:

Semi-Vegetarians–They eat fish and occasional poultry dishes.

Lacto-Ova Vegetarians–They eat no meat, but do consume dairy products and eggs.

Vegans–(pronounced VEE–guns) Probably the least common group today, they're what most of us call total vegetarians. They don't eat any animal products whatsoever.

Vegetarians tend to weigh less, have lower cholesterol levels, and higher fiber intakes. With diabetes, these benefits alone may be worth eating this way. However, for people with diabetes, vegetarianism can also be a good way to control calories and protein intake (those with kidney problems take note). Plus it feels like you can eat more when you have a vegetarian diet, since you "bulk up" with a lot of filling fresh fruits and vegetables.

Even if you want to change your diet just a little bit, it's a good idea to see a Registered Dietitian. Your dietitian can make sure your new diet has the nutrients you need to grow, mature, and meet your calorie requirements without upsetting your blood sugar balance. Be aware that any change in diet, even if it's a healthy one, can affect blood sugar control. This can make the change frustrating, but working with a specialist can help you over the hurdles so you don't feel like your attempt was a flop.

> **Bottom Line:** You have lots of options for healthy eating, but make sure that what you do is for the right reasons and that you're doing it safely.

FOOD FADS

You may have friends who suddenly get into doing new things because they think it's cool. These fads pass quickly—remember Star Wars, Cabbage Patch Dolls, and torn sweatshirts? The only reason to do something is because you want to do it or believe in it. We know, sometimes it's hard to resist doing something because you think it'll make you look cool, but the truth is that people respect individuality. Dare to be different!

Food fads are what people eat when it's what everyone else is doing. Or they have a mistaken notion it will make them stronger, thinner, or healthier. Sometimes a food fad can be unhealthy because it deprives your body of important vitamins, minerals, and protein it needs for growth. If you're thinking about going on a particular diet, first check it out with your dietitian.

SPECIAL OCCASIONS AND PARTIES

Most of the time parties and special occasions can be managed with a little bit of forethought and planning. With the smaller and faster blood testing meters, it's pretty easy to test blood on the run. Then you know what to eat, when to take your shot, and how to manage a special occasion food.

There are probably times when diabetes becomes a pain in the neck, though. When you're invited to a party or friends decide to get together, diabetes can smack you with a reminder that you can't always do what you want, when you want, without thinking ahead. If you ignore your diabetes, you could pay the price by running too low or too high and feeling lousy.

Of course, being prepared isn't always easy. Say you're out with friends who decide to go out to dinner, but you forgot your insulin and syringe. Or you take less insulin, planning to go swimming in the evening, but when you get to the pool, it's closed! Or you might be hanging out with a friend who asks you to sleep over. Once again, diabetes gets the better of you when you have to say no because you don't have your stuff along. Besides, you can't sleep until noon on Saturdays without getting high blood sugar and you don't want to get up at 9:00 and wake everyone up. We still have times when it feels like diabetes gets in the way, even though we know it doesn't have to.

When you were younger, your parents probably prepared you for special events and holidays. They might have called to let people know you had diabetes and brought along diet sodas, fruit, and special sugar-free desserts so you wouldn't feel left out.

Now that you're older, you choose the parties and things you want to go to. There are some that happen every year no matter what (like holidays, birthdays, the Fourth of July, etc.). So how do you come prepared for these fiestas? Most of them have certain foods associated with them, some of which might be in your plan and some of which might not.

Here are some suggestions for making things easier:

Plan Ahead–
Find out what the activities and menu will be like wherever you're going. Usually all it takes is a phone call! Restaurants will even be happy to let you know their specialties, specials for the day, or the kinds of dishes they can make for you. Airlines accept requests for vegetarian, diabetes, or low–cholesterol meals (just call 24 hours in advance). Even if you're going to someone's house, call and ask

what they're planning on eating and offer to bring something to help out. Look up the carbohydrate content of some of your favorite fast foods so you're prepared when you go to Burger King or Baskin-Robbins. With your doctor's approval, you might, when out with friends, keep a pre-filled syringe of Regular insulin with you, so if they decide to stop for a snack, you can cover yourself for your favorite foods!

Keep Diet Soda Handy–

It might be helpful to keep a six-pack of your favorite diet soda around. If you're going on one of those beloved family car trips, load up beforehand. Jean often packs cans of diet soda when she travels, just in case she can't find them wherever she's going.

At a recent family wedding, Sue discovered that no diet soda was available at the bar at the reception. Taking the bull by the horns, she drove to a corner store and bought a six–pack. She took it back to the bar at the reception in a brown paper sack and asked them to simply serve it to her when she approached the bar. No problem! In fact, the bartenders said they would make sure that they had something sugar-free at their next event! (Everyone else kept asking for Sue's diet soda, too.)

Substitute Special Foods For Those In The Meal Plan–

If you can fit special foods into your normal meal plan, so be it! Talk with your doctor, nurse, and/or dietitian about how to do this before you try it. For example, you can let your parents know that you'll be subtracting some starch and protein from dinner in order to have pizza later at the football game. With your doctor's approval, you could take less short–acting insulin at dinner and cover the pizza later with the difference in the short–acting insulin. If you count carbohydrates, you can use your usual insulin–to–carbohydrate ratio to account for the pizza. Approximately one unit of Regular insulin can cover 10 to 15 grams of carbohydrate eaten. Make sure to test your blood sugar level so you know how much insulin to take if you're adding extra food to your usual pattern.

Pick Five To Six Holidays A Year Where You Can Eat What You Want–

Everyone needs to take a breather once in a while, but frequent testing is required so you know how your blood sugar took that pumpkin pie! It may also require extra insulin to keep blood sugar in range. Check with your diabetes educator if there are holidays that you'd like to be able to do this. The problem with frequently covering extra food with extra insulin is that it is easy to gain weight.

Account For Exercise/Dancing–

For events like school dances, proms, tennis matches, or soccer games, try to figure out ahead of time how active you'll be. If you're more of a stander, chatting and eating at dances, no big deal. But if you love dancing, you might want to plan ahead. A little more exercise can lower blood sugar a lot! (Sallie finds that just 30 minutes of shopping at the mall—not the most invigorating activity—can send her blood sugar plummeting!) The key again is more frequent blood sugar testing.

WHAT ABOUT DIETING?

Few people (especially girls) survive the teenage years without going on at least one diet. We've all sworn to live on rabbit food or go jogging every day in order to look like the models on the cover of *Glamour* or *GQ*. (Sooner or later, we also realize that as long as we feel good about ourselves, it doesn't matter that we don't look like Cindy Crawford.) There's so much information on counting fat and watching weight and wearing certain kinds of clothes that it's easy to start taking it all a little too seriously. You may be willing to sacrifice activities you enjoy, friends, or even school itself because the number on the scale isn't where you want it to be. However, pounds on a scale are pretty meaningless. In fact, what's more important these days is your percentage of body fat. A model and a ballerina may look exactly the same size and wear the same size clothes, yet the ballerina weighs 10 pounds more because her muscles are heavier.

Often, young women with diabetes find that running higher blood sugar allows them to control weight. Insulin is a storage hormone. When your blood sugar level is in range most of the time, or when you change your insulin and it improves, you may notice a small increase in your weight.

Although controlling weight this way might work for the time being, just like fad diets sometimes work, the real questions here are not whether or not you lose the weight, but instead: 1) is it safe? and 2) can it provide a long-term answer? **When it comes to using high blood sugar ranges to manage your weight, the answers to both of these questions is NO!**

Think about what might be lost as a result of this behavior—you might not be able to concentrate on tests at school or even the lectures, which could lead to poor grades. You'll feel tired and sick most of the time, so you might not be able to participate in your favorite sports and activities. You'll find that you have other undesirable side effects such as bad breath, frequent urination, thirst, and poor vision.

Leah, a young woman, learned what a bad idea it was to try to let her blood sugar run high. At first, she found that it was more difficult to keep blood sugar up than down! She ended up eating a lot in order to keep the glucose up and had times where her weight would increase before it would drop again. Then she tried not taking insulin and became so sick she ended up vomiting and having high levels of ketones in her urine. (She missed the dance where she was going to wear the dress she was dieting to get into!) The revelation for Leah was, *"I was trying to control something I really didn't understand well. I felt terrible and unhealthy."*

So what can you do if you're tempted to use bizarre ways to control your weight? How can you work through your obsession with counting calories, grams of fat, and pounds on the scale? Eating disorders occur for many reasons. Sometimes your quest for a skinnier body is a mystery to everyone but yourself. It will most likely require a team approach to help you sort out all of the forces at work here. One suggestion is to see a counselor, psychologist, or social worker (who is also a CDE if possible). A registered dietitian can also be a big help in trying to work through your best food choices and figuring out a calorie level and exercise program that will keep your weight stable.

There are actually a lot of ways to control your weight without the guilt, control, and obsession that dieting often produces. In fact, many people find they do better if they aren't so strict with themselves when they're trying to lose weight. The more you try to avoid the refrigerator, the more you'll hear it beckoning you to try some chocolate ice cream. The best thing to do is face the fridge and choose yogurt instead of ice cream. Exercise is another way to keep weight stable, as long as you continue to eat the calories you need for growth and development. Relaxation time built into your day often relieves anxieties about eating, since many people use food as a way to relax. And changing your own thought patterns about food (there's no such thing as a good or a bad food!) is a helpful way to deal with some of the decisions you make about eating.

To get back to Richard's Rules, there are times when you eat more and times when you eat less. So you already *know* how to eat less! What is it that makes it possible for you to eat less and make healthier choices sometimes, but not at other times? Build on what you know has worked well for you in the past and will make eating as small an issue as possible for you in the future!

FOOD GUIDE PYRAMID

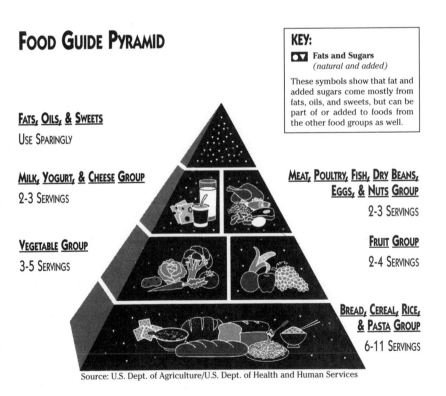

KEY:

▨ Fats and Sugars
(natural and added)

These symbols show that fat and added sugars come mostly from fats, oils, and sweets, but can be part of or added to foods from the other food groups as well.

FATS, OILS, & SWEETS
USE SPARINGLY

MILK, YOGURT, & CHEESE GROUP
2-3 SERVINGS

MEAT, POULTRY, FISH, DRY BEANS, EGGS, & NUTS GROUP
2-3 SERVINGS

VEGETABLE GROUP
3-5 SERVINGS

FRUIT GROUP
2-4 SERVINGS

BREAD, CEREAL, RICE, & PASTA GROUP
6-11 SERVINGS

Source: U.S. Dept. of Agriculture/U.S. Dept. of Health and Human Services

CHAPTER 3
TIGHTENING UP CONTROL

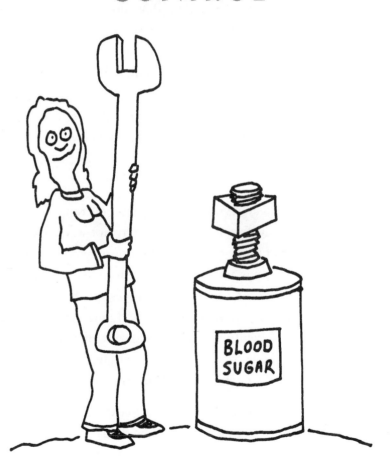

BLOOD
SUGAR

In Control

The Diabetes Control and Complications Trial (DCCT), which ended in 1993, looked at whether tight control of blood sugar levels helps prevent or delay complications of diabetes. According to the study, it does! So all your hard work will definitely pay off in the long run.

"So what?" you might say. "I'm already doing the best I can, I don't need more pressure and guilt to do more!" (OK, so you didn't say it, but maybe you were thinking it!)

Well, like it or not, what you do today could catch up with you tomorrow. Even though you think you're doing just fine, every little bit closer you get to your target range can help your chances for a healthy future. We believe that even though the future may seem pretty far away, it **IS** worth some extra trouble, although we know that it's hard (especially when you're a teen). It's tough enough for us, diabetes wizards that we are, to juggle diabetes with husbands, kids, a dog, jobs, travel, and book writing! So what can we do differently?

If your blood sugar levels are in your target range and your HbA_1C is within your target limits, you may not want to do anything differently. But if you have room for improvement, there are probably a lot of things you can do to help move toward your goals. Some of these may be major changes, such as changing insulin types, number of injections, or scheduling. Others may be smaller changes, like waiting 30 minutes after taking insulin to eat or substituting pretzels for the cookies that give you high blood sugar. The first step is deciding you want to make a change.

What steps are reasonable? (We're not advising you to give up TV or clean up your room or anything like that!)

1. Talk to your doctor or health care team about your concerns. (See Chapter 10 for help).

2. As before, don't forget the little steps. Always take your insulin, test blood as often as possible, and use test numbers to improve things. Little changes such as just making sure you wait 30 to 40 minutes after taking insulin to eat can help.

3. Think about moving toward multiple daily injections (three or four shots a day) or an insulin pump.

4. Take it as a challenge to get in the best control possible.

> **Bottom Line:** The lower you can get your HbA₁C without having a lot of severe low blood sugar problems, the better your chances are for a long, healthy life.

You may want to consider these options:

MULTIPLE DAILY INJECTIONS (MDI)

Many people in the DCCT study were on three or four shots a day, or an insulin pump. On more shots a day, a long–lasting insulin such as Ultralente gives you a steady amount of insulin between meals. (Some folks used two shots of NPH in the same way.) Then you take a fast–acting insulin (Regular) to cover meals and snacks. The idea here is to try to mimic what your body should be doing: putting out a little insulin all of the time and extra insulin when food is eaten.

Ron, a 17-year-old high school junior, decided to try multiple daily injections a year ago. *"At first I thought it would be too much trouble to take four shots a day. I didn't want to do it, and didn't want to have to think about it. But when I started, my blood sugars smoothed out right away, and the funny thing was I felt like I was in control of things for the first time in my life! I could make these decisions and control my blood (sugar) based on what was going to happen in the next four hours. So I could decide if I wanted a big lunch or not, and cover it with insulin. I could cut back if I had hockey practice, etc. I use an insulin "pen" to take my lunch dose and nobody thinks twice about it."*

Pros of MDI:

- There's a little more flexibility in meal timing and scheduling.

- You have extra chances to adjust insulin to bring a high sugar down, exercise, or make meal alterations.

- There's a better chance for improved control of blood sugar.

Cons of MDI:

- You must do blood testing before taking insulin. (Otherwise, you don't know how much to take!)

- You have to carry insulin supplies wherever you go, just in case you need them.

- You may be more likely to have low blood sugar.

PUMPING UP

An insulin pump is about the size of a beeper and has a syringe full of Regular insulin inside it. The syringe is connected to a little tube (or catheter) that has a needle at the end of it which is about the size of an insulin needle. One type of needle has a thin covering of Teflon. When you push it into your abdomen or hip tissue, you pull the needle out and the Teflon tube stays there for a few days until you pull it out and put in a new one. The Teflon is soft and bendable, so it's pretty comfortable. You may have seen one in some of the diabetes magazines. Ask your doctor or nurse to show you one if you're interested. Both Jean and Sue have pumps and like the flexibility they have in food choices and timing of meals.

Sue finds that dressing up is sometimes a hassle, especially when she wants to wear something a little flashier. When she puts on a little black dress, a pump sticking out of the side isn't exactly the look she's going for. Avoiding this problem usually means having to disconnect the pump for a short time, or going back to shots for a few hours. It might seem like a high price to pay for fashion, but then is any price too high? (Jean thinks so—she usually finds a place for her pump somewhere and doesn't buy tight clothes!)

PROS OF PUMP THERAPY:

– There's more flexibility in your life. Meals don't have to be as "on schedule" as with other ways to manage diabetes.

– You can raise or lower the hourly amount of insulin to adjust for sickness, exercise, etc.

- You may take extra doses (called a "bolus") when needed for extra food and you don't have to take an injection.

- You don't have to carry syringes and insulin with you everywhere you go.

- People think you're athletic when you say you're "pumping up" and will ask you how many miles you did that day.

CONS OF PUMP THERAPY:

- Having hardware stuck to your body all the time can become quite annoying.

- It isn't cheap (ask your team about cost comparisons).

- It's all too easy for your body to make ketones if for some reason you don't get the insulin, which can happen if there's a leak.

- You can get infections at the needle sites.

- You should disconnect for contact sports.

- You sometimes get stopped at airport security when they ask you to "put it in the little box" as you pass through scanning. (It takes some time to explain that you can't disconnect it!)

There's a lot to think about when choosing which way to go. You need to find out what works best for you.

> **Bottom Line:** Little changes in diabetes care can go a long way to improve blood sugar levels.

ALTERNATIVES TO EXCHANGES

At some point you may have used (or could still be using) a meal plan based on exchanges. Most people use the American Diabetes Association/American Dietetic Association Exchange Lists for Meal Planning, which have been used for eons to help people regulate food types, meal times, and how much they eat. The idea is to balance the way your insulin works. The problem is that meal planning based on exchanges doesn't always fit YOUR schedule. Today, with the results of the DCCT study and people taking insulin and testing more often, it may be better to match insulin to food. Fitting diabetes into your daily life is usually more successful than trying to adjust your life to diabetes. You need to show diabetes who's boss! These days, the best way to go about it is to set your schedule yourself and let your diabetes care team adapt your diet and insulin to meet your needs. After all, no two people are alike.

One of the more popular meal plans used in the DCCT was "carbohydrate–counting." You may want to think about trying this, if you haven't already. (Talk with your doctor, dietitian, or diabetes educator first.) The idea is to count the number of grams of carbohydrate you'll have at each meal or snack and take a certain amount of insulin to cover that carbohydrate intake. Going back to Jean's Dairy Queen ice cream cone, it doesn't so much matter what you eat as long as you adjust for carbohydrates. The other bonus is that you can have a snack along with everyone else, whenever you want, as long as you cover it. You can even play with the carbohydrate content of your meals from day to day (it doesn't always have to be exactly the same) as long as you take more or less insulin if the carbohydrate is more or less.

In Control

Where to start with this? If you're familiar with exchanges, you might know that one starch, one skim milk, and one fruit exchange all contain about 15 grams of carbohydrate. Many diabetes specialists feel that one unit of Regular (short–acting) insulin can cover 10 to 15 grams of carbohydrate pretty well. Or if you don't want to refer to exchanges at all, just check the food labels for grams of carbohydrate in a food, and you can base your insulin needs on that.

So let's return to Frank. Let's say he's heading to a football game that will end around 10:30 p.m. and then his friends are planning to stop at McDonald's afterwards. Frank eats dinner at 6 p.m. before doing his homework and showering for the game. His blood sugar is 105 (5.8 mmol/L) before dinner. His favorite choices at McDonald's are a quarter pounder with cheese and medium French fries. He looks up the carbohydrate content and finds that a quarter pounder with cheese is 34 grams and medium French fries are 36 grams of carbohydrate (total=70 grams). At the restaurant, he tests again and his blood sugar is 152 (8.4 mmol/L) (his target range is 80 to 160 [4.4 to 8.9 mmol/L]). Since he's in range, he figures he can have the burger and fries by taking the right amount of insulin to cover these. If his ratio is one unit of Regular insulin to 10 grams of carbohydrate, he takes seven units of Regular insulin about 30 minutes before his late night McDonald's snack.

Since blood sugar levels can drive teens and everyone else to the edge, being able to adjust as you go along can be very helpful. It's always a good idea to talk to your health care team about ways to do this. You'll probably find that they can give you the basic information to start with, but you'll be the one letting them know which foods, activities, and ratios work the best (or worst) for you. So don't be afraid to experiment, you never know what will hit the jackpot.

You may find that it's often not worth your effort to eat some things. For example, Sue found that cornflakes cause a large blood sugar rise for her. Even though it took her nearly a day to get readjusted after this, she thought she'd try it again just to make sure! The same thing happened (of course). So much for cornflakes in the morning. Interestingly, the same thing happened with nacho chips, corn tortillas, and cornbread. These are all products made from degermed cornmeal—something Sue found out after a couple of hit–or–miss meals and with a little detective work. In fact, people with diabetes should try to find out what effect different foods have on their blood sugar. One guy found that a couple of Hostess Twinkies raised his blood sugar from a normal level of 102 to 268. We've heard this referred to as the "Twinkie tolerance test." The next time, he covered his Twinkie with five units of Regular insulin and went from 110 to 180 (6.1 to 10.0 mmol/L)—better, but still not enough insulin. Finally he tried six units and found that his "Twinkie allowance" of six units of Regular insulin works quite well and keeps his blood sugar levels in his target range.

Of course, it's not a great idea to be eating a lot of extra food all the time and then taking a lot of extra insulin to balance it. First of all, you'll gain some major tonnage just like anyone else. Second, it's hard to guess the effect of certain foods on your blood sugar. But if you know how to manage different foods, eating on special occasions doesn't have to be a big deal. You may also find that once you give yourself permission to have these other foods, you may not want them so much anymore!

In Control

CHAPTER 4

THINGS THAT GET IN THE WAY...

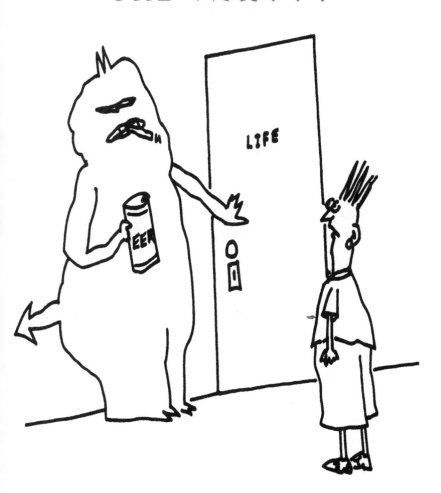

There are many reasons why people turn to alcohol, drugs, or other destructive behaviors. Some think it will help them escape their daily problems. Others think it will help them fit in. Whatever the circumstances or reasons, the plain truth is that there is no such thing as "safe" alcohol, drugs, tobacco, or sex—saf*er* but not 100 percent safe. Regularly taking these risks is a sign that you may need some counseling help to take better care of yourself.

DEPRESSION

Do you ever feel that getting up in the morning is like pulling yourself out of quicksand? Or that you never have the energy or will to DO anything? Maybe you feel like your friends or family never understand what you're going through. Depression affects thousands of teenagers today. No one ever said being a teen is easy. You have advice coming in from all directions and so many expectations to live up to (including your own) that maintaining your sanity is often an accomplishment in itself. And when you have diabetes to add to the list of peer pressures, homework, job responsibilities, chores, guy/girl problems, and trying to have fun, it can really get you down.

Drowning your sorrows in an alcoholic stupor isn't a new concept (even if it is to you). It's been put through the old feel-better test and failed time and time again. Not only does it make you feel worse emotionally, but physically it's not a joy ride for your body. Plus you could end up doing things you wouldn't normally do and will feel awful about later. Smoking or using chewing tobacco is another way that teens try to relieve stress. Unfortunately, this doesn't work either. You won't end up feeling better and you increase your chances of getting cancer. It's VERY important to talk to a parent, teacher, or other adult if you're having any of the following problems:

- poor grades in school
- a lot of tardiness or absences from school
- aches and pains that keep you from doing what you want to do
- poor concentration
- loss of interest in friends, sports, or activities
- crying all the time
- sleeping all the time, not being able to sleep, or awakening early
- feelings of sadness or hopelessness
- changes in appetite
- thoughts of suicide

If you think you might be depressed, there are counselors in most schools to help. You can also talk to a parent, doctor, clergy member, or other adult. There are medications your doctor can prescribe to help you fight depression. You don't have to take it lying down.

> **Bottom Line: There's help out there if you need it!**

SUBSTANCE ABUSE

Teens can use drugs and alcohol for a long time before parents and others even have a clue that there's a problem. Kids can turn to drugs or alcohol for many reasons. The following can put you at greater risk for developing a problem:

- If you have a mother and/or father who has abused alcohol or drugs

- If you have a brother or sister who has abused alcohol or drugs

- If you have a grandparent who has abused alcohol

Have you said the following to yourself or others? If so, it's a sign that you need to get some help: "I may be using alcohol/drugs, but no more than my friends do. My drug/alcohol use is no big deal—I can stop whenever I want to."

Using these substances on a regular basis can lead to physical and/or psychological addiction. You may feel worthless or like the world and you just don't get along, and alcohol or drugs offer an escape. But escape is only temporary. Your problems will be back in your face the next morning, along with a hangover and bad feelings about how you acted. Substance abuse can also cause friend, school, sleeping, and diabetes problems. That can lead to even more substance abuse. The cycle just keeps going. It's critical that you talk to a parent, guidance counselor, member of the clergy, doctor, nurse, or other adult to help you get back on track.

It's important for you to know the effects of drugs and alcohol on diabetes. Drugs and alcohol can have varied effects on blood sugar. One problem is that the high and low feelings you may get from drugs and alcohol can mask the signs of low blood sugar.

ALCOHOL

Drinking alcohol is a hazard to your health, especially when driving is involved, as everyone knows. But it also doesn't exactly do wonders for your diabetes. Alcohol has no nutritional benefit. It's processed in the liver like a fat, so it's usually counted in the diet as a "fat exchange" if you're using an exchange diet.

Alcohol can also make you forget to take your insulin, or help you forget how much you ate while you were drinking.

Once Sue was planning to go to a wedding and she asked her doctor about drinking alcohol. His advice was, "If you haven't started drinking yet, don't." Not a bad idea.

One of the problems with drinking alcohol for someone with diabetes is that it can cause low blood sugar by blocking the release of sugar from the liver. Sometimes this effect may not occur until hours after drinking. When you have diabetes, it's especially important to eat when you drink alcoholic beverages. (We've heard about people who have diabetes and have also been drinking who have been jailed for public drunkenness when, in fact, they were having signs of low blood sugar. Alcohol on their breath, confusion, and lack of coordination made them appear to be drunk.)

Obviously, it's best for your diabetes if you choose NOT to drink at all. However, if you do drink, here are some guidelines:

- Have your medical ID with you.

- Choose light beer, light wine, or white wine instead of liquors. Alcohol can be watered down by mixing it with diet soda, club soda, or water. Read the amount of carbohydrates on the label.

- Don't drink on an empty stomach. Drink slowly and sparingly.

- Make your own drink when possible. (Don't take any chances!)

- Limit yourself to two drinks.

- Check blood sugar often after drinking alcohol—especially if you're exercising.

- Make sure there's someone with you who knows you have diabetes and knows the signs and treatment for low blood sugar.

TOBACCO (CIGARETTES AND CHEW)

Tobacco hurts anyone who's using it. When you have diabetes, the risks are multiplied. Nicotine, the drug in tobacco that is addicting, affects blood pressure, the heart, and blood vessels—as does diabetes. So when you put the two together, they jack up the risks of developing diabetes complications such as heart, blood vessel, and kidney diseases.

Smoking can also hurt your ability to perform in athletics. When you smoke, the blood in your lungs can't pick up oxygen as easily, so you get winded a lot faster. The use of tobacco also causes stained fingers and teeth, cigarette burns, cancer of the gums or nose (smokeless), smelly clothes and breath, and an emptier wallet.

Some teens have switched from cigarettes to "chew" or snuff, thinking it cuts the risks of lung cancer. However, with chew and snuff the effects of nicotine in the body are sometimes even greater than with cigarettes, because more nicotine may actually absorb into your system all at once. Again, blood vessels are affected, which can cause high blood pressure, and, in someone with diabetes, lead to kidney disease.

If you decide to quit using tobacco products, the signs of "withdrawal" from tobacco can be confused with signs of low blood sugar. Some of these signs are drowsiness, headaches, irritability, hunger, and anxiety. These can also be signs of low blood sugar. Blood testing, in this case, is VERY important.

MARIJUANA

Regular users of marijuana can be at greater risk for using other types of drugs. Not only is the use of this as well as other drugs illegal, but they can lead to serious mental, emotional, and physical problems. When you have diabetes, the problems can be magnified.

Marijuana usually causes an increase in appetite, so if you're eating more, grazing on food, or nibbling all day, blood sugar levels can be high. On the other hand, if it's getting in the way of remembering to eat regular meals, blood sugar levels may run low.

Other drugs such as cocaine and barbiturates can, like marijuana, have varied effects on diabetes control. In some cases drugs will lower blood sugar and in other cases, raise it. Using drugs on a regular basis can cause you to have personality changes such as becoming withdrawn, secretive, angry, and sleepy. Usually grades will drop and friends will change (not for the better). The chemicals in marijuana can also irritate your breathing passages and cause coughing. If you use any of these drugs in the morning, it's a sign that you're probably hooked. Use of cocaine is also an advanced sign of substance abuse.

> **Bottom Line:** If you're regularly using drugs, alcohol, or tobacco, you're headed for trouble. Get help now!

STRESSFUL TIMES

Stress causes the release of the hormone adrenaline (or epinephrine).* This is the same hormone that causes you to feel shaky and sweaty and makes your heart race. Adrenaline also raises blood sugar levels.

---

* *Adrenaline (epinephrine) is a hormone released in times of stress or excitement that can raise blood sugar levels. It also causes some of the symptoms of low blood sugar levels, such as sweating, shakiness, and a racing heart .*

In Control

If you're under a lot of pressure, chances are you also have high blood sugar. Some teens notice that blood sugar levels might run high during finals week, after breaking up with a girlfriend or boyfriend, or after a few sleepless nights. Family disruptions such as parents divorcing or a death in the family are other examples. Your body is also under stress when you're sick with a cold, flu, or infection. Increased ketones can be an effect of stress if your body isn't getting enough insulin.

What stresses out a friend may not necessarily be stressful to you. Figuring out what makes you a basket case probably isn't the hardest task in the world. Unfortunately, sometimes there isn't a lot you can do about it. (You could become a monk, but that probably isn't much of an option. Actually, that may be stressful in its own way.) It's important to treat high blood sugar levels with extra insulin no matter what the reason, and try to prevent the stress if you can.

John says he's uptight when he comes home from school, so he uses exercise to help him relax: "I just go out for three or four miles, and I'm fine." Sharon, on the other hand, takes a nap: "I know if I can just rest for a half hour, I'll feel pulled together when I wake up." There are other people that use stress reduction techniques such as listening to music or prayer to help them relax. (Some people also swear by yoga!)

> **Bottom Line:** Figure out what stresses you out and try to prevent it. If blood sugar is high, make adjustments.

CHAPTER 5
SEXUALITY AND BIRTH CONTROL

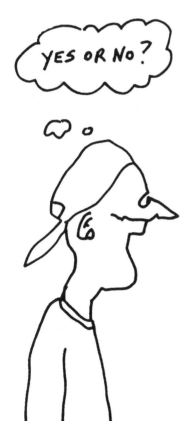
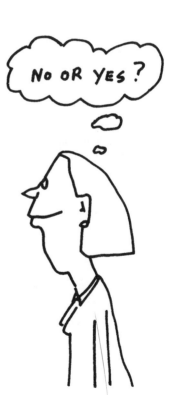

What's Right For Today?

Sexuality doesn't just mean "going all the way" or "doing the deed." It includes all your feelings as a sexual guy or girl. It's a process that begins when you're born and continues throughout your life. Your sexuality is a part of you, and it includes your thoughts, feelings, and values as well as your body, arousal, and intercourse.

When you have diabetes, not only do you have to worry about the usual things everyone else does, but you may also be curious about how your disease affects your sexuality—or if sexuality affects diabetes. This stuff isn't easy, and you'll probably face some big decisions.

What's Right For Your Health And Diabetes?

Sexuality isn't only about sex itself, but also about how you view yourself. You might think of yourself as a sexy super-stud or as someone who will never be more than a buddy to the opposite sex. Body-image and self-esteem have a lot to do with the way you feel. Sometimes diabetes becomes an easy scapegoat for image problems.

We've heard people blame their diabetes because they're too fat, too thin, or too short. But don't even try to pin the blame on diabetes for zits, snoring, cavities, and split ends—it just won't fly. Plus, looking for something to blame doesn't accomplish anything, and diabetes probably has nothing to do with most of these concerns. What does matter is self–confidence. How can you expect someone else to like you if you don't even like yourself?

GROWING AND CHANGING

You're very unlikely to make it through your teenage years without going through puberty. It's pretty much inevitable. But life after puberty isn't easy either. You have to deal with how you feel about yourself and how others feel about you. If you're the type that's always being asked out, you might have to work a little harder at controlling your sexuality. If you're someone who never seems to be asked out, you have to find ways to show people the good stuff you're made of.

Your growth and maturity depends on certain hormones in your body. Everyone matures at different times, although girls tend to do so before boys. You never know when it's going to hit you, but wishing for it to happen isn't going to help a whole lot. You may know some friends who began to grow and develop around age 12, and others who were 16 when it happened.

In females, the first changes may be the beginning of breast development, hair under the arms or in the groin area, and a growth spurt. Girls will have reached most of their adult height by the time of their first period. (Average age is 12 1/2 years.) Males usually start their growth spurt a little later than girls and may notice an increase in the size of their testes and penis, and start having wet dreams. This is perfectly normal and precedes growth.

Hormones are generally responsible for your sexual feelings and for that day when the opposite sex stopped being gross. (Cooties ceased to exist at this point.) Your self–esteem (the way you think about yourself as a sexual person) can be based on the way you look or the way you think you look to others and yourself.

Diabetes won't hold back your growing and developing unless you don't have enough insulin during your growth years. Your body needs insulin to feed the cells so you can grow and mature. You may have noticed that your doctor takes your height and weight measurements when you have an appointment. This is to make sure you're growing on schedule. If you're lagging behind, you may need more tests to figure out why.

DEVELOPING RELATIONSHIPS

Diabetes can sometimes affect both how you feel about yourself and your sexual relationships. During the tender teen years, you might find yourself experimenting with relationships (sexual and otherwise). If you aren't having the greatest experiences, it probably won't do wonders for your self-esteem. On the other hand, when you're in control and doing well, it can spill over into other areas of your life.

This is also a time for trying out relationships with all sorts of different people—giving people a chance who aren't like any of your other friends. This is part of finding out who you are and the kind of people you want to hang out with. When you have diabetes, finding out how other people react to your disease is also part of the bargain.

Most of the time, friends will take their cue from you as to how they should react to diabetes. If you're positive and upbeat and sometimes joke about it, they probably will, too.

BIG DECISION #1:
TO BE (OR NOT TO BE) SEXUALLY ACTIVE.

Many teens today are deciding they *aren't ready* to have sex. This is a smart choice if you can make it, because you'll avoid risking AIDS, sexually transmitted diseases (STDs), and pregnancy. One 16-year-old told Jean that she decided to abstain because she thought having diabetes was enough to handle and she didn't want to have to worry about anything else. A mature decision! It's not always that easy, though. It's pretty hard to say no when your friends are all having sex and someone is pressuring you to do it. Many people think it's always wrong for teens to have sex, but the decision to have sex should be your own. Ask yourself if you're really ready to handle it, not if your friends, boyfriend, or girlfriend think you *should* be.

When you're making a decision, it can be helpful to talk to someone who's older and wiser (for instance, the ever-enlightened adult). A parent, doctor, nurse, clergy member, or teacher can be helpful if you have questions or just want to chat about it. There is no foolproof way to be sexually active and be completely safe from serious infections and pregnancy. However, if you've given it some serious thought and think you're ready to have sex, you'll need to make BIG DECISION #2.

> Bottom Line: The decision to have sex should be your own.

Big Decision #2:
The choice to be protected.

As stated before, there is no such thing as completely safe sex, but unprotected sex is just plain stupid. You may be exposing yourself to HIV (a virus that causes AIDS—and death), other diseases, or pregnancy. Contraceptive foam for females and condoms (otherwise known as rubbers) for males, when used together properly each time you have sex, can be effective in avoiding an unwanted pregnancy or a sexually transmitted disease.

Family Planning Clinics and others can help you with information and guidance on birth control methods or other sexual problems. There's no cost for attending a clinic, and visits are confidential. To find a clinic in your area, contact your local hospital or ask someone on your health care team.

How to Use Contraceptive Foam:

Buy a brand that says "contraceptive foam" or "spermicide" on the package. Read the instructions that come with the foam. (Keep them for future reference.) Be sure the foam's expiration date has not passed. Follow the package directions precisely. The following are general guidelines.

1. Shake the can 20 times before using. (This makes sure that the spermicide mixes with the foam, and that there are a lot of bubbles.) Fill the applicator with foam.

2. Use one or two applicators-full of foam right before sex. (Read the directions ahead of time to know how much.) Put the applicator high up into the vagina and push in the plunger.

3. Foam protection lasts about 30 minutes. Use another dose if more than a half hour has passed between the first dose and intercourse.

4. Wait at least 8 hours after the last time you had sex if you want to douche.

5. Wash the applicator with soap and warm water.

6. Keep a spare container on hand because there is no way, with most brands, to tell when you're getting low.

7. Use more foam if you're going to have sex again.

The foam works because spermicide kills the sperm made when the male ejaculates (or comes) inside the woman's vagina. Foam doesn't guard against HIV. It works better to prevent pregnancy when it's used with another method of birth control, such as condoms. Condoms are put onto the man's erect penis just before intercourse. Condoms prevent the sperm from being released into the vagina.

Everyone's heard of AIDS these days, but some teens think they won't get it if they live in a wealthy suburb or only have unprotected sex once in a while. The truth is that it can hit everyone. Over one–fifth of people with AIDS are in their 20s. Because there's a lag time between the first contact and the symptoms, most of these people were probably infected with the virus as teens.

Other sexually transmitted diseases are also common. Some of these are syphilis, gonorrhea, chlamydia, and other viral infections. These diseases can lead to infertility, cancer, and other major health problems. Also, you could get genital ulcers from unprotected sex, and such infections put you at a greater risk of developing AIDS.

The other reason for using condoms and foam is to prevent pregnancy. However, women who decide to become sexually active might, with their doctors advice, decide to take birth control pills or use other forms of birth control. (See "The pill and other birth control methods," page 64.)

How to Use a Condom:

1. Use a condom every time you have sex.

2. You or your partner should put the condom on the penis before putting it into the vagina. Roll the edges all the way to the bottom of the penis. Leave about one–half inch of empty space at the tip, or buy condoms with nipple tips to hold the semen.

3. After sex, hold on to the condom as you withdraw the penis. Be careful not to spill semen near the vagina. Withdraw the penis immediately after ejaculation because loss of erection can cause the condom to slip off (and pregnancy can result).

4. Store condoms in a cool, dry place. Don't keep your condoms in your wallet because body heat can cause the rubber to break.

5. Spermicidal cream, foam, or jelly (not petroleum jelly or Vaseline) can be used to lubricate the outside of the condom.

6. Check the condom for holes or tears before you throw it away. If you find any, or if it has torn or come off in the vagina, quickly insert contraceptive foam or jelly.

(See other methods of birth control on page 64.)

> **Bottom Line:** There's no such thing as completely safe sex, but you can make it safer by using foam and condoms each time you have sex.

If you haven't protected yourself for any reason or if the condom tore or came off (or you've been raped), the "morning after pill" will often prevent pregnancy. Your doctor or clinic can give it to you upon request and can tell you how to use it properly.

MALE CONCERNS

Some teens with diabetes wonder if it will affect their sexual performance. The answer is "no" unless you've had diabetes for many years and have complications. If your blood sugar is running very high all of the time, however, it may affect your sex drive, just because you're dehydrated, tired, and not feeling well.

Most men with diabetes need to do frequent blood testing to find out how sexual activity affects their blood sugar levels. Because of the physical exertion, some men may need to eat more or take less insulin, just as they do when they exercise. On the other hand, others may find that their blood sugar levels run high because of the release of adrenaline into the system. (See "Stressful Times" on page 51.)

After years of diabetes, some people develop neuropathy. This usually happens when nerves become affected due to years of high blood sugar levels. When the nerves affected go to the genitals, men may have trouble having or keeping an erection. Clogging of the blood vessels leading to the penis can add to the problem. The penis won't become or stay hard. Impotence can have many causes besides the complications of diabetes. Keeping blood sugar levels in range can do a lot to prevent this from happening.

If you're worried about the threat of impotence, you're not alone. Keith told us:

"One of my strongest memories as a teenager was listening to the lectures on impotency caused by having diabetes. I remember listening to lectures in which they stated that men with diabetes wouldn't be able to perform sexually. At that point in my life, 99.9 percent of my thoughts, both while sleeping and awake, centered around the topic of sex, so this was information that I was very concerned about! Later, when I studied diabetes in more detail, I learned of the importance of keeping blood sugars as close to normal as possible, and that impotency can be treated. The anxiety diminished but the interest remains strong!"

FEMALE CONCERNS

Women may also wonder if diabetes will affect their sexual performance or pleasure. Again, as is true for males, diabetes shouldn't affect sexual functioning except in the case of dehydration or a vaginal yeast infection. If sex is painful, see your doctor.

VAGINAL YEAST INFECTIONS

Women with diabetes are more prone to vaginal yeast infections because high blood sugar helps the yeast to grow and can change the pH (acidity) of the vagina. Wearing tight or constricting clothing, such as swimsuits, spandex, or nylon underwear can add to the problem. Antibiotics can also cause an overgrowth of yeast.

Signs of vaginal yeast infections can include itching, pain, and/or irritation in the genital area. There may also be a thick white or yellow discharge. There are several over-the-counter medications that you can buy to treat these infections, but you should consult your doctor the first time you have symptoms to make sure of the diagnosis. Also, see your doctor if the treatment is not working. Wearing cotton underwear and looser fitting clothing, using unscented sanitary pads during your periods, and wiping front to back after a bowel movement can help prevent yeast infections.

MENSTRUAL PERIODS

Diabetes and your period can affect each other in different ways. If your HbA_1C is running high, you may find that your periods aren't regular. On the other hand, you may find that your blood sugar level may be high around the time of your period. It can happen a week or so before the flow starts and is due to changes in female hormones. These hormones cause insulin to not work as well. Also, many women report getting the munchies around the time of their period, so they eat more than usual. If you notice your blood sugar level running high before or during your period, talk to your doctor about changing your insulin doses during those days.

PREGNANCY

Pregnancy can be very successful today for women with diabetes and their babies. But it takes a lot of work to control the blood sugar and it takes a lot of planning ahead. When you're pregnant and have diabetes, both you and your baby can be at risk for big problems. If you already have complications from diabetes, sometimes pregnancy can make them worse.

One of the most important periods in the development of a baby is the first few weeks of life, before you may even know that you are pregnant. If the mother's blood sugar levels are not in excellent control during this period, the baby might not grow correctly or may have other problems. The risk to the baby continues throughout pregnancy, and there's some research suggesting there may be lifetime effects. This is why it's very important to control blood sugar levels tightly before and during pregnancy. Pregnancy can also cause blood sugar levels to go crazy. You might be very low at some times during the pregnancy and high at others.

> **Bottom Line:** Get your blood sugar levels in range before you get pregnant. If you think you're pregnant, see a doctor immediately.

THE PILL AND OTHER BIRTH CONTROL METHODS

Oral contraceptives (birth control pills or "the pill") contain female sex hormones. The pill works by creating a steady hormone level that sends a message for the ovaries not to release an egg each month. When there is NO egg, there is NO pregnancy. If there were an egg, it would also have trouble attaching itself inside the uterus because of the changes in the lining of the uterus caused by the pill.

If you follow the directions and don't skip taking them, the pill can be over 99 percent effective in preventing pregnancy. If a woman has high blood pressure, heart problems, liver disease, or cancer, or has had a stroke or blood clot, she should not take the pill. When you have diabetes, you should be able to use the pill for birth control, but it's very important that your doctor follow your progress closely.

There are some side effects from taking birth control pills. Most of these will go away after your body adjusts. Some of the possible side effects are: small weight gain, headache, breast tenderness or enlargement, nausea, mood changes, fluid retention, and decreased menstrual flow. When you have diabetes, birth control pills may make your blood sugar levels rise, causing you to need more insulin.

Smoking cigarettes increases the risk of high blood pressure, blood clots, and heart problems. Since diabetes and tobacco also increase these risks, it's NOT a good idea to have diabetes, smoke, AND take birth control pills. Your doctor probably won't let you use the pill if you smoke. Other types of birth control are also available with different levels of effectiveness. You may want to talk to your doctor about whether these would be good choices for you.

BARRIER METHODS:

METHOD: Diaphragm

DESCRIPTION: Soft rubber cup that fits over mouth of uterus.

EFFECTIVENESS IN PREVENTING PREGNANCY: 85%-97%

DRAWBACKS: More effective when used with spermicidal jelly. Must insert in advance or interrupt lovemaking.

METHOD: Sponge

DESCRIPTION: Absorbs/acts as a barrier to sperm.

EFFECTIVENESS IN PREVENTING PREGNANCY: 90%

DRAWBACKS: Must insert in advance or interrupt lovemaking. The sponge should stay in for 6 hours afterward.

HORMONAL METHODS:

METHOD: Depo-Provera® (sterile medroxyprgesterone acetate suspension, USP)

DESCRIPTION: Injection of hormone that works for 3 months to prevent pregnancy.

EFFECTIVENESS IN PREVENTING PREGNANCY: 99.5%

DRAWBACKS: Can cause irregular or heavy bleeding during your period.

METHOD: Norplant® System (levonorgestrel implants)

DESCRIPTION: Hormones released from device implanted under the skin.

EFFECTIVENESS IN PREVENTING PREGNANCY: 99%

DRAWBACKS: Must be implanted by doctor and can raise weight.

LESS RELIABLE METHODS: (NOT IDEAL FOR ANYONE)

METHOD: Rhythm

DESCRIPTION: Avoid sex 3 days before and after ovulation.

EFFECTIVENESS IN PREVENTING PREGNANCY: 60%-85%

DRAWBACKS: Must know when ovulation occurs.

METHOD: Withdrawal

DESCRIPTION: Remove penis from vagina before ejaculation.

EFFECTIVENESS IN PREVENTING PREGNANCY: 75%

DRAWBACKS: Hard to stop and/or control. Also, some semen may be ejaculated before orgasm.

METHOD: Temperature Monitoring

DESCRIPTION: Monitor basal temperature to determine ovulation and avoid sex during the time the temperature rises.

EFFECTIVENESS IN PREVENTING PREGNANCY: 60%-85%

DRAWBACKS: Another thing to measure, inaccurate.

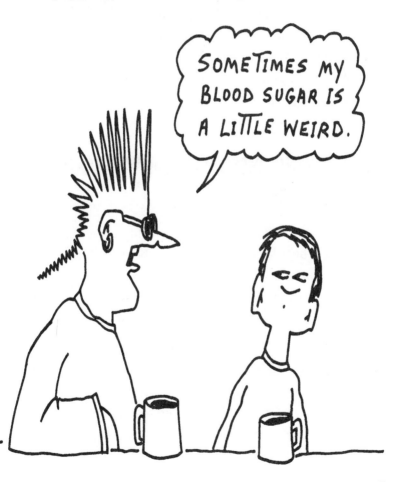

Life would be pretty boring without other people in it. Some people you work with, others you live with, some you're intimate with, and others you only say "hi" to when you pass them in the hall. Of course, you don't exactly go around advertising your diabetes, so you have to decide who you want to tell and who you don't think has to know. And the perfect time to share your little secret just never seems to pop up. How do you tell them?

Just as you have different levels of contact with people, you probably need to have different ways of telling them about your diabetes, if you tell them at all. For example, does the grocery store clerk or the crabby neighbor down the street NEED to know about your diabetes? You might want to think about the people you interact with on a regular basis and ask yourself where they fit into the following categories:

People Who Need To Know About Your Diabetes:

People who fit into this category might be your parents, college roommates, best friends, girlfriend or boyfriend, teachers, coaches, supervisors at work, and/or relatives you may spend a lot of time with. They should have some understanding about your diabetes schedule and all you need to do to take care of yourself.

Those who NEED to know are people you'd count on to help you through a crisis with your diabetes that you might not be able to handle by yourself. For example, they understand low blood sugar and how to treat it. You should teach them how to give you glucagon if you ever need it. These are the people you feel closest to and feel comfortable telling about your diabetes.

Beth Ann told us about one experience she had:

"When I got to aerobics, even though I've never had low blood sugar that I couldn't handle myself, I knew that somebody in class should know that I have diabetes—just in case. I thought the instructors were the most logical people to tell, but I thought they might worry that I'd have a problem. Also, even though I've always been open about having diabetes, I was hesitant to tell them because we were just getting to know each other, and I wanted them to think of me as Beth Ann, not as the student with diabetes.

"Telling them turned out to be no problem at all! In fact, a few positive things happened: First, I learned that, as instructors, they're expected to know if anyone in the class has diabetes. One instructor was interested because her daughter's friend had diabetes. I explained what my possible needs might be to one, and another already understood my needs pretty well. No one treated me differently; they saw that someone with diabetes can be healthy and active!"

PEOPLE FOR WHOM IT'S NICE TO KNOW ABOUT YOUR DIABETES:

People who fit into this category might be relatives you don't see often, people who have invited you to a party, and some of your classmates. These people probably spend less time with you but may be in a position to help out in case of low blood sugar or be around at insulin time.

In some cases, it's not absolutely necessary but it is a good idea to let people know you have diabetes. For example, when you're going out of town for an away football game, it's smart to let the bus driver or chaperon know you have diabetes. Or when you go to someone's house for dinner and hear the food will be late after you've taken your insulin, you might tell someone. People will usually be helpful if they know what your needs are. These people can help prevent a fiasco.

"Bean" is a young guy who uses an insulin pump to control his diabetes. At first he was a little worried about what he should tell people about this weird object that was now attached to him. *"When I got my pump, I decided to tell my best friend, Pip, all about it,"* he says. *"I showed him how I hooked it up, how to turn it off and on, and anything he should do for me in case of an emergency. I told my other close friends that it was a thing I wore to control my blood sugar. I told everybody else that it was a walkman!"*

PEOPLE WHO DON'T NEED TO KNOW ABOUT YOUR DIABETES:

People who fit into this group might be the grocery store clerk, your mailman, most of the people at your school or college, and the gas station attendant. These people really have nothing to do with your schedule or diabetes care.

When Sue first got her insulin pump, one of the nurses at the hospital thought it was a cute fashion accessory attached to her belt. Sue was about to go through the whole routine about how it's a device used to regulate blood sugar . . . blah, blah, blah, and then she thought better of it. There was really no reason that the nurse had to listen to a long, detailed explanation. So Sue just let her think it was a fashion statement.

When Jean was exercising, a weight–lifter came over and asked if that little box attached to her shorts was a "newfangled pedometer" to measure her miles. She explained, "No, it's my insulin pump!" He laughed and replied, "Yeah! Now, what is it really?" She could have used her precious exercise time to explain, but decided it just wasn't worth it, so she laughed and moved on. (What some people don't know won't hurt them!)

DATING AND MARRIAGE, THINGS TO THINK ABOUT:

Telling the person you're dating about your diabetes can be a dilemma. You might wonder if they'll think you're flawed in some way or if the idea of syringes and low blood sugar reactions will make them queasy. It might take a while to get up the guts to tell people who need to know about your diabetes. Since you'll probably end up spending a lot of time with a boyfriend or girlfriend, it's important to be open about diabetes as soon as possible.

However, it's sometimes hard to tell your friends about diabetes. Most of the time it's best to get it out of the way right away. Usually, people take their cues about how to react from you. So if you have a positive, matter–of–fact attitude about diabetes, so will almost everyone else. On the other hand, if you're embarrassed or bummed out when you talk about it, others might feel uncomfortable.

In Control

Sue freely admits to having made some mistakes when she dated. In fact, her mother ended up breaking the news to her fiancé after she became very sick with the flu, a whole year after they'd been dating! Sue's mom asked her, "Just when were you going to let Bill know about your diabetes?" Sue said she was just "waiting for the right time." (To this day, Sue can't figure out how she kept it from him for so long.)

If a friend held out on you for a long time, how would you feel? Sue realized that it really wasn't fair putting Bill at risk for finding out by accident. In fact, Bill accepted it with no problem. "So that's why you only have a diet coke after the movies while I stuff my face!" he commented. Acceptance (with or without approval) is a true way of showing someone you care.

Jean, on the other hand, told Jim about her diabetes the first time they met. The next day, he went to the university medical library and read all about diabetes. They were engaged about six months later!

Some people ask their boyfriend or girlfriend to follow a schedule and pretend they have diabetes for a while before getting married. They do things like take shots, wear a pump, do blood glucose tests, eat a timed and portioned meal, etc. They get to know the thrill of living with your special friend, diabetes. It's important to help them understand what you have to deal with day in and day out. Sometimes this helps them come up with great ideas that you haven't thought of for helping you get through tough spots! You might even want to get your best friends to try it out.

On the flip side, even though friends can understand part of what it's like to have diabetes, they'll never completely know what it's like. In the back of their minds, they realize they can quit in a week or two and be just fine. (It's like when you used to pretend you were blind by putting a bandanna around your eyes, always knowing that you could just take it off.) Your friends don't have to worry about complications and know that their experiment will end. They won't be doing this stuff for the rest of their lives.

One teen told us that he sometimes used diabetes to break the ice when meeting someone new: "It can lead to great conversation and give you a feeling for the intelligence and sensitivity of your date!" (We're not sure about the intelligence part, but this was his screening method!)

> **Bottom Line:** There are people who need to know about your diabetes, some for whom it's nice to know, and others who you'll choose not to tell.

In Control

CHAPTER 7

ON YOUR OWN

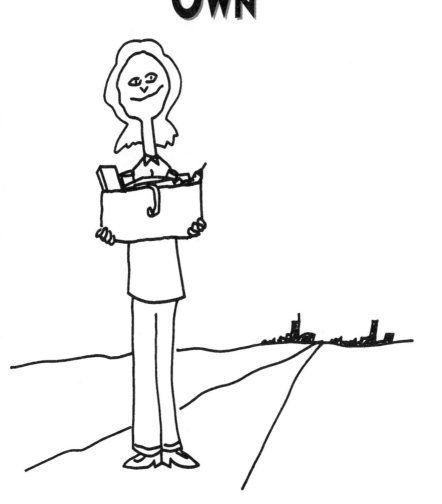

Trying to figure out what to do with the rest of your life can be a big headache. Whether you decide to go to college, technical school, or jump right into the work force, you have some big decisions to make. You might want to ponder the best way to fit diabetes into the career you choose. Whatever that may be, remember that diabetes doesn't have to be the focal point of your life.

WHAT ARE YOUR LIMITS?

There are very few things you can't do because you have diabetes. You can't be in the military, you can't fly a commercial airplane or drive a school bus, and you shouldn't be a construction worker who works on tall buildings (insurance companies won't cover you because of the risks of low blood sugar—dizziness isn't really a plus.) In the past, scuba diving wasn't recommended, although there are now scuba camps for people with diabetes who want to give it a go! Aside from these few exclusions, there's very little you can't do with your life. Jobs that have night rotation schedules are tough, but you can find ways to do it and still keep blood sugar levels in range. The idea isn't to find a job that can accommodate diabetes, but to fit diabetes into whatever life you choose for yourself. There are ways of dealing with all kinds of lifestyles.

Dan is now a physician who thought he was going to have to drop out of medical school because his blood glucose levels were bouncing up and down from his crazy work schedule. Dan was also a competitive figure skater, which made it even harder. His blood sugar levels would be high all day and low all night. After experimenting with different ways of solving the problem, he discovered that an insulin pump gave him the flexibility to cut the amount of insulin he got during and after skating, and to increase his insulin for days he had high blood sugar or wasn't eating right.

When Meredith went to college, she had the worst possible class times her first semester (as do many lowly freshmen). She started with an 11 a.m. class and ran straight through until 3 p.m., then had more classes from 4 to 7 p.m. She missed lunch most days and dinner three days a week. Then she'd sleep late in the morning, skipping breakfast—not the best schedule for managing diabetes. After talking to her doctor, Meredith decided to try going to a multiple daily injection routine in which she took long–acting insulin first thing in the morning and short–acting Regular insulin before meals and snacks. She says her blood sugar levels are still up and down a lot, but better than before, and she likes the flexibility.

NEGOTIATING DORM LIFE

When you're leaving home for the first time, diabetes gives you a lot to think about. Who to tell, how much to tell them, buying/having the right kind of food on hand, getting a refrigerator, maintaining diabetes supplies, safely disposing of syringes and lancets, managing parties, and teaching someone how to use glucagon are all things to consider (in addition to those few other things new college students have to deal with). No problem, right? Actually, it doesn't have to be a big deal if you plan in advance. If you're living far from home, you'll need to find a local doctor who can work with your usual doctor to care for your diabetes while you're at school.

In Control

With all the things to pack and buy for college, diabetes supplies probably aren't your biggest priority. Eric, a university sophomore, shared his revelations about college:

"My whole life, the Supply Fairy just magically knew when I was low on stuff. Like when I'd be down to three or four syringes, another box would just reappear in my closet. Well, it was a rude awakening when I discovered that the Supply Fairy didn't visit me in my dorm. I had to run out of stuff a few times (always at the most critical moments) before it hit me that I was going to have to take care of this myself. My roommate, as it turned out, had to take a lot of medicine for allergies, so we'd alternate trips to the drug store."

Another thing to think about is how you're going to get rid of your sharps and lancets. Milk jugs and empty soda bottles work OK. However, it might be best if you can get a commercially prepared "sharps" box. These boxes have to be disposed as medical waste. The student health service office on campus will usually collect and dispose of these boxes. Safety is key here. You need to protect people from accidentally pricking themselves and make sure that the syringes are destroyed and can't be reused in the wrong hands.

When you're making friends in college, feeling different because of your diabetes isn't unheard of (although most people feel different or weird because of something). Sarah, now a junior, talked about her fear of managing diabetes in a new situation, and how it all turned out:

"I was so afraid that my diabetes would get in the way of making friends at college. I was embarrassed, feeling different, and wasn't sure who to tell. What happened was that because of the setup of the dorm, the fire codes, and a cafeteria in our

building, we weren't supposed to have little refrigerators in our rooms. But because I really needed to have one for snacks or missed meals, I got special permission to have a fridge. At first people sort of reacted with surprise that I could have it. They didn't care about diabetes, but my room was the most popular place to meet on my floor. Everyone would come in to visit and put something in the fridge!"

Most college students will teach their roommate and maybe one or two other friends about the signs, symptoms, and treatment of low blood sugar. They'll need to know:

– usual symptoms you have (shaky, disoriented, sweaty, etc.)

– first line of action (sugary soda, glucose tabs, gel, juice)

– second line of action (how to give glucagon)

– where supplies are kept

– who to call/phone numbers

George didn't tell his new roommate, Stan, that he had diabetes right away and actually hid it amazingly well. One day, though, Stan walked in right as George was giving himself his shot. Both sort of jumped and Stan went a little crazy until it all got straightened out. (Having a heroin addict as a roommate wasn't such a pleasant idea, apparently.) From then on, George was upfront about his diabetes with his roommate and close friends.

Consider the benefits of telling your teachers or profs about your diabetes. Our friend Gary, a professor, had this experience:

"A student (whom I knew to have diabetes) was taking a final exam. I noticed that she seemed distracted and wasn't looking well. I asked her if she was having difficulty, but she assured me that she was just tired from pulling an all–nighter studying for my exam and another test later that same day. Five minutes later, I literally caught her as she was falling out of her chair. I was able to treat her because I knew of her diabetes. If I hadn't known, the result might have been more of a problem."

On The Job

Whether you're working to make a living or to make a little extra cash in school, you may want to think about how diabetes fits into your work schedule. The Americans With Disabilities Act guarantees that you're entitled to take the necessary steps to provide proper medical care for yourself in the workplace. Employers must provide "reasonable accommodation" to workers with disabilities, and diabetes does qualify as a disability. This means your employer must allow you to take care of your diabetes while on the job. This could mean letting you take breaks to follow a meal or snack schedule or providing a place to keep diabetes supplies handy.

You may need time to test blood sugar or treat a low blood sugar. You'll probably want to tell someone where you work (a supervisor or trusted co–worker) about your diabetes in case of an emergency.

CHAPTER 8
THIS, THAT, AND OTHER STUFF

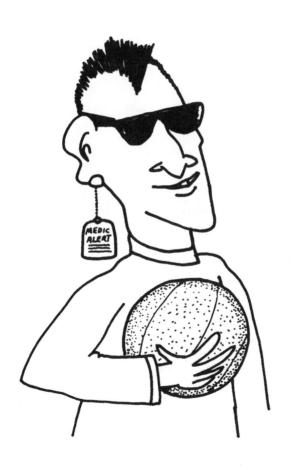

In Control

It's a good thing you don't have too much to think about, right? Sure, you may feel like you have a ton of responsibilities and choices to make. But look at it this way, you're already totally used to making decisions around the clock because of your diabetes. So maybe you've got an edge over your friends. Decisions about college, sex, sports, careers, etc., might be easier for you because you've had so much practice. Then again, maybe not. It's OK to ask a friend or special adult to help you sort through a problem or help you make a tough decision.

MEDICAL ID

Some people think wearing a medical ID is like wearing a billboard that says, "I have diabetes!" However, the fact that you're wearing an ID doesn't advertise anything. People wear these for contact lenses, penicillin allergies, bee sting allergies, asthma, and all kinds of other reasons. Michelle said that "instead of using the cheesy old line 'I have something I think you ought to know,' you can use your ID to tell your date about diabetes."

Having a medical ID doesn't mean you have to look like a dork. Janice, 16, commented, "I saved my babysitting money to buy a gold ID. I figured if I'm going to wear it all the time, it might as well be a pretty piece of jewelry." On the other hand, there are also colorful nylon wristbands that come in great colors, are inexpensive, and look super.*

In the case of an accident or severe low blood sugar, it's extremely important that medical personnel know about your diabetes so they can treat you properly. As the old saying goes: Don't leave home without it!

*Colorful Nylon Diabetes ID Bracelets are available from Major Medical Supply, 1675 18th Ave., Greeley, CO 80631.

Other sources for medical IDs are:

Medic Alert Foundation U.S.
P.O. Box 1009, Turlock, CA 95381-9009, 1–800–432–5378

Goldware
P.O. Box 22335, San Diego, CA 92192, 1–800–669–7311

S&L Goldsmiths
P.O. Box 56, Lavon, TX 75166, 1–800–229–9829

Westags, Inc.
P.O. Box 108, Flourtown, PA 19031, 1–800–BECAUSE

Identifind
Rt. 4, Box 420A, Canton, NC 28716, 1–704–648–6768

Life Alert
P.O. Box 68527, Portland, OR 97268, 1–403–258–0822

SPORTS

Sports are great ways to get in shape, hang out with friends, and have a blast. If you can find one that really turns your cranks, stick with it. Of course, some people find that playing a lot of different sports can help keep life interesting. Whatever you play, staying active is key. While it doesn't always make diabetes control better, it's still good for you.

When you play sports, you'll need to make some adjustments in your insulin and/or food. If you're usually pretty active, it will probably require less adjusting than if you're a couch potato who has suddenly decided to go in-line skating! Also, different types of sports will have different effects on blood sugar levels. For example, an aerobic exercise like cross country running, swimming, or basketball can cause faster drops in blood sugar levels than shot–put, wrestling, or weight training.

In Control

When adjusting your insulin around sports, talk to your diabetes educator to help you plan how to do it. What you do will depend on:

- the time of the sport (after school vs. evening, etc.)
- the intensity of the sport (cross country vs. sprints; time on the bench vs. continuous play)
- the kind of insulin regimen you're on (two shots vs. more)
- how tight your usual control is (how much room you have to drop blood sugar levels)
- your usual response to exercise

Another question that comes up is "What should I do about those 4:30 to 7 p.m. practices?" Baseball, wrestling, swim team, and other athletic practices are often during the usual dinner time. Again, this will have to be worked out on an individual basis. Part of the decision to take your insulin early or late will depend on the types of insulin you're taking and when. It will also depend on your usual insulin schedule and your blood sugar numbers. For example, some teens who take three shots will take less Regular insulin at 4 p.m., eat dinner, and take NPH at bedtime. Others may want to eat a heavy snack before exercise, then take their insulin, and then eat dinner. What's best for your blood sugar levels and your schedule needs to be worked out by you and your doctor.

A late drop in blood sugar is common after exercise. Sometimes this post–exercise drop can happen up to 24 hours after strenuous exercise. This is why you can have low blood sugar the night after an active day. You may wonder why, since your blood sugar was OK at bedtime and you ate a snack. What happens is that your body cells are still taking up blood sugar at a faster rate after you exercise—and it can hit you late! Many people will also need to cut back their long–acting insulin in the evening on active days.

You may also want to pay attention to where you take your insulin injections, since your activity can affect how quickly it's absorbed. For example, if you use your leg for your shot and then go running, or your arm and then play tennis, absorption of the insulin may be much faster, causing low blood sugar.

Participation in some sports can encourage you to do things that may not be in the best interest of your diabetes (or your over-all health, for that matter). This could happen in wrestling, when sometimes people do extreme things to "make weight," or during events when coaches may encourage you to try "carb–loading."

Gary, our friend the university professor, shared this story:

"I had a male student who was a member of the varsity wrestling team. He found an "effective" way to get his weight down (a tough task for wrestlers) by letting his blood sugars ride high. He would stop taking insulin until he started pro-ducing ketones and losing weight. He did this until one day he temporarily lost his vision. Mike had to rethink his lifestyle."

When you're participating in various sports, you'll find that each sport has its own "culture." Often, part of belonging to that culture may include eating or avoiding certain foods and using sup-plements (such as protein drinks, sports drinks, or vitamin/miner-al supplements).

Just like adjusting insulin is specific to the sport and you, so will your food adjustments need to be for you and you only. At this point, the most helpful person on your diabetes team will probably be a dietitian. She/he can help you figure out the benefits of certain types of sports drinks and supplements. Although your diet needs to be designed specifically for you, it's important to note a couple of things:

- Many supplements and beverages are expensive. Make sure that your usual diabetes care doesn't suffer as a result of putting dollars into something less beneficial. For example, Marc thought that extra protein was a must as he prepared for body building. He stopped buying glucose strips so he could purchase a special protein formula (for about $60 a month)! He wasn't even sure what the formula did to his blood sugar because he wasn't testing as much. When he talked to his dietitian, she showed Marc how he could almost double his protein intake every day with just a couple of dairy–based snacks (yogurt with crackers or two bowls of cereal at night).

- Many of the protein and sports drinks on the market contain large amounts of fast–absorbing carbohydrates and sugars. These will need to be accounted for in your meal plan and adjustments made in your insulin. On the other hand, the best liquid for fluid replacement is plain old water. Drink two cups for every pound lost during a practice or game. Moderate dehydration can make blood sugar numbers appear higher than they really are, so drinking water isn't such a bad idea. If you need a fluid with carbohydrate to balance a low blood sugar, full–strength fruit juices are the best choice. If you need a source of fluid and carbohydrates to get you through an activity, try diluting fruit juice half–and–half with water and drink 1/2 cup every 10 to 15 minutes during the activity.

Your dietitian can determine your need for a vitamin or mineral supplement. By analyzing your diet on a computer, a dietitian can see that you might need to eat certain foods for the vitamins or minerals deficient in your diet. If you don't like the foods she comes up with, she may suggest that you take general multivitamins or multiminerals.

ALL-NIGHT ACTIVITIES

When you stay up all night to cram for a test, dance the night away, play a sports event (like all-night bowling), or go to a fund raiser (like a dance marathon), routines can get pretty screwed up. What to do usually depends on the situation at the time. If you're up all night doing something, your body will obviously burn more calories than when you're asleep. If you're dancing or exercising, you may need to eat something every couple of hours to get more calories. Another option, which can be used along with more food, is to cut your longer-acting insulin at dinnertime and cut or eliminate the short-acting insulin as well. Adjustments may have to be made for the next day, since you'll probably sleep in and not be as active. Again, longer-acting insulin taken in the morning may need to be decreased and short-acting insulin may need to be cut down or eliminated. Testing urine for ketones can help you decide whether you need more insulin.

Prom time can be one of the most fun and exciting times of your life. (Although, there are plenty of prom horror stories out there.) You don't want to blow it by not taking care of yourself and not feeling good enough to enjoy it! Going to the prom or doing other all-night activities doesn't usually help blood sugar control, but sometimes you just have to sacrifice a little control to live your life. By paying attention to what's going on with blood sugar, you can usually get through it with no problem.

Driving

The word on the streets is SAFETY, both for you and everyone else on the road. You never know when a traffic jam will delay a meal or snack. Here are safety guidelines EVERYONE with diabetes should follow when on the road:

– Always test blood before getting behind the wheel.

– Test blood every two hours while driving.

– If you think you might be low, always pull over immediately and test or eat.

– Always carry a fast-acting sugar and crackers in the glove compartment.

– Drive with a friend whenever possible.

– Carry extra food for long trips.

– Don't leave your meter, strips, or insulin in the car longer than necessary. They are sensitive to heat and cold.

– Wear your medical ID.

And these, of course, apply to everyone (with or without diabetes):

– Always wear your seat belt.

– Never drink and drive!

SUMMER

The biggest change in diabetes care for summertime may be that you're more active and require less insulin. Your schedule may be different too, since many teens tend stay up later at night (usually as late as possible), and sleep later in the morning (usually as late as possible). This might mean some serious adjusting of insulin schedules and amounts.

What happens when you have a pump and want to go to the beach or pool? With a pump, laying out on a beautiful sunny day won't affect the quality of your insulin. One pump type is waterproof so you can even wear it in the pool, lake, or ocean, and the other has a waterproof case you can use for water sports. However, some people like to switch to multiple daily injections for stays at the beach or pool. Then you can stay outside and swim spontaneously and not worry about taking care of the pump hardware. (But you might want to worry about wearing sunscreen—have you heard about the size of the hole in the ozone layer?)

While on shots, Sue chose injection sites that didn't bruise as much (the abdomen) so it wouldn't show when she wore a swimsuit. In fact, she says her control is usually so much better while on vacation that her doctor has given her a prescription for a "permanent vacation!"

In Control

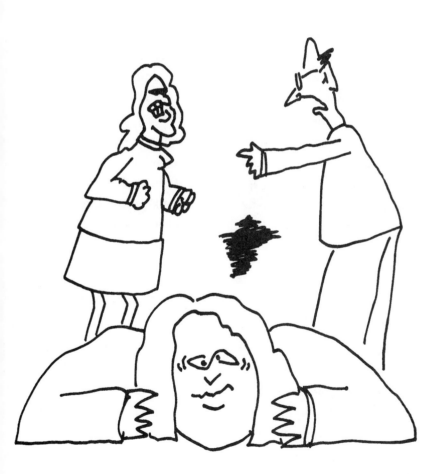

CHAPTER 9
SMOOTHING THE WAY

In Control

Maybe we should call this section "Soothing the Way." We don't know if there's such a thing as a smooth route to diabetes care, but family members definitely need some soothing after the diagnosis. Think back to the day you were diagnosed—how did the people around you react? Their actions may help you understand their feelings about diabetes in general and you in particular!

Often, family members feel they're to blame for causing your diabetes. You may be tempted to blame them too. It's important to understand how others view your diabetes. What they see and feel may not be what's actually happening, and that can cause problems.

Sue clearly remembers her mom's dismay and guilt after Sue was diagnosed with diabetes. Her mom cried all the way to the hospital. She blamed herself for passing along family genes that gave Sue diabetes and worried that maybe she hadn't fed Sue right over the years or that there was something she could have done to prevent it. She also wished the diagnosis was hers and not Sue's. But Sue's mom obviously hadn't done anything to give Sue diabetes. While she knew that on an intellectual level, it took her a long time to get over the feeling that maybe she could have done something to prevent it. This feeling isn't uncommon among parents (as you probably know).

On the other hand, there are times when diabetes (or YOU, because you have it) gets blamed for something when it has nothing to do with what's really going on.

Mr. and Mrs. Bennett argued a lot about their daughter Julie's diabetes, which turned into a focal point for their problems. But Julie's blood sugar level was generally in her target range, and she appeared to follow the management plan her diabetes team had given her. At one visit, she began to cry. As her educator talked to Julie, she found out that Julie's parents fought at home about a lot of different things.

What was REALLY going on? Julie's parents had been having problems for a while, and were starting to blame it on the diabetes. Instead of confronting the problems with their marriage, it was easier to blame the diabetes and Julie, since it avoided dealing with the real source of their pain. Julie was feeling like her diabetes was to blame, but it wasn't the real problem! Things got better after they went to family counseling sessions and started to work on the real issues.

The Brown family had little money and seven kids, so things were pretty tight. The costs of supplies, insulin, and testing strips for their daughter Judy were a real problem, since the other kids needed coats, shoes, and school supplies. Her parents struggled with how to get Judy treatment without favoring her over the other kids. Her dad argued about how many times a day she needed to test and how much insulin was actually required. At home, he would get upset at the dinner table when Judy had to have larger helpings of food to meet the meal plan. Then she stopped testing or took smaller amounts of insulin so it would last longer because she felt guilty. Not surprisingly, diabetes control was not going well.

The real issue was that Judy felt like it was her fault when her dad got angry. However, her dad wasn't really mad at all; he was frustrated because he didn't have enough money to provide for his family and take proper care of her diabetes. When the diabetes team discovered what was going on, the social worker gave the family some places where they could apply for extra help for diabetes care.

If this sounds familiar, it's very important that you talk to your health care team to help your family find some solutions. Both of these situations show that diabetes is complicated AND involves the whole family. The best way to deal with the emotional, financial, and physical aspects of diabetes is to get them out on the table.

> **Bottom Line:** If your family is having conflicts about diabetes issues, seek counseling.

HELPING BROTHERS AND SISTERS

Often brothers and sisters feel that diabetes is used by the person who has it to get what they want (including attention). As the one who has diabetes, you shouldn't feel guilty about extra attention you may get. After all, it's reassuring to know your parent will be there to help you or any brother or sister who faces challenges. But you may need to decide what you can do for yourself and how others can help you. Sometimes, brothers and sisters can also worry too much or feel overly responsible for diabetes care. You should let them know that they aren't responsible for taking care of you, but they can help out once in a while.

> Looking back, Marian says, *"Growing up with a sister with special needs was difficult at times, but overall it has helped me to be more sensitive to each person's uniqueness. If I could have changed things for her, I would have in a second, but I'm grateful for the many ways she has enriched my life."*

Your brothers and sisters can be great supporters (when they want to be). As long as they understand what you need to do, they can help you stay on track.

CHAPTER 10

MAKING FRIENDS WITH YOUR DIABETES TEAM

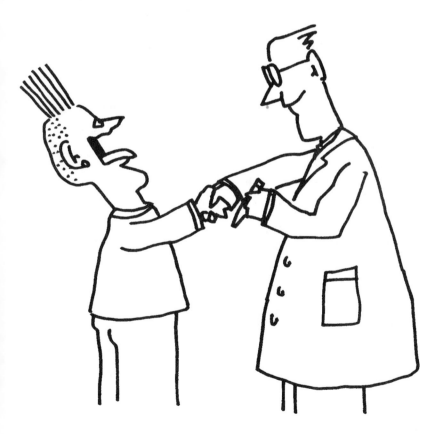

Why Have A Team?

When you have diabetes, every area of your life is affected, including your family. It's next to impossible for one person, your doctor, to handle all the issues that come up for every patient. That's why it's important to look for a team of experts in diabetes care. You're also on the team (as a VIP member, of course). The whole team works together to solve problems and make life with diabetes as smooth as possible. In this book, we've suggested using your health care team to support and guide you along the way. However, what should you do if there aren't qualified recruits in your area?

Sometimes there are team members available, but they just aren't centralized in one location. For example, your doctor's office may not have a dietitian or diabetes educator available at the time of your appointment, but they may know or work with such people in your area or at a local hospital. You may have to ask your doctor for a referral. (See Resource Organizations on page 107.)

If your team isn't centralized in one place, *you* may have to do the work of contacting them and/or putting your team together. What's most important, however, is that you feel comfortable working with them. If you don't feel like you can talk to them, keep looking until you find someone you work well with.

A Visit To Your Team

How would you describe your health care team, including your doctor? Strict, authoritative, iron-handed drillmasters? Or easy-going, soft-spoken, accommodating helpers? All right, so maybe these are extreme examples, but you can probably come up with your own adjectives.

When you see your health care team, do you break into a cold sweat? Does it make you think about doing things that you'd never considered doing before? Or do you enjoy going because you get support for what you ARE doing and they help you work through difficult situations? Do they nag you or boost you up?

How about neither? Your health care team is a service that you're paying for. Instead of thinking of them as a second set of parents or friends, consider them paid consultants. Now think about this: Would you pay someone a lot of money to give you advice and then NOT follow it? What's wrong with this picture? Why is it that the very people who are there to help us are the same ones we often feel the need to lie to and fool?

What's the best way to use your team to make your life easier and your health the best it can be? They're there to give you the best of their knowledge and experience. (Just remember that they have lives, too.)

It requires a team approach to treat diabetes, but you're the captain here. You set the tone, you steer the ship—after all, it is your diabetes and YOU live with it 24 hours a day! But you're not alone with that responsibility. Just like any sports team, all the players have to work out your game plan and execute the plays. Only then can you come through with a score. That way, not only can you share the spotlight of a perfect goal, but you also have someone with whom you can share the blame when decisions don't turn out so great.

> **Bottom Line:** When something doesn't work out, everyone learns from it. Go back to the drawing board with your team! It doesn't necessarily mean you did something wrong.

SOME TEAM MEMBERS MIGHT BE:

Certified Diabetes Educator (CDE)

This nurse, dietitian, pharmacist, social worker, exercise physiologist, physician's assistant, psychologist, or doctor is a licensed health professional who has taken a national exam on diabetes education and care. His or her job is to educate you about diabetes so that you can learn to manage it and prevent complications.

Endocrinologist/Diabetologist

This doctor (MD) will probably be the one you see most often. Endocrinologists are specialists in hormones, such as insulin. Diabetologists have a special interest in or are experts in the care of people with diabetes. Their role is to coordinate your plan of care.

Social Worker

This health professional (MSW/LISW/LSW) can give you information about diabetes services and medical care and help you find groups to support your diabetes management. A social worker can also help you explore ways of getting financial help and give you counseling support for the emotional tugs that diabetes sometimes causes.

Registered Dietitian

This health professional (RD) can help you work through food–related issues, provide you with your own personalized meal plan, offer recipes and resources for a healthier diet, and help you keep your weight controlled during periods of improved blood sugar control and hypoglycemia. Seeing your dietitian as often as you see your dentist is important, because as your life circumstances change, you'll need adjustments in calories, timing of meals, and insulin.

Registered Nurse/Nurse Educator

A nurse educator (RN) can become one of your closest allies in keeping diabetes in tune with your needs. A nurse will probably be the first person who teaches you about diabetes, how to do your blood sugar readings at home, and how to give insulin. As you live with diabetes, this person can guide you through all the usual and unusual situations you have to work the diabetes into (pizza parties after the football game, prom, studying late for tests, illness, traveling and vacations, camping, etc.). A nurse educator can make adjustments in your testing schedule, help you set goals for blood sugar control, and help coordinate things with other members of the team.

Exercise Physiologist

This health professional (MS) is helpful for active teens who want to include exercise in a daily routine and participate on sports teams at school. He or she can plan the best times of day for exercise and set up a plan for testing blood sugar around exercise periods. Exercise physiologists can help you become physically fit while keeping your diabetes management under control.

Ophthalmologist

This doctor (MD) specializes in eye diseases. After five years of insulin-dependent diabetes, everyone should have their eyes checked by this doctor at least once a year.

In Control

Counselor/Psychologist/Behavioralist/Psychiatrist
This doctor (PhD or MD) is an expert in behavioral science and can help if you're having difficulty adjusting to or coping with diabetes or other family concerns.

Nephrologist
This doctor (MD) specializes in kidney diseases. If someone with diabetes starts to develop kidney problems, they'll go to this doctor.

Podiatrist
This doctor (DPM) specializes in foot care. He or she can help with problems such as foot infections, ingrown toenails, sports injuries to the feet, and foot surgery when needed. You might need to see this doctor regularly, especially if there's a problem with circulation or nerves to the feet.

You
You're also a member of the team. Your team involves coaches, players, and cheerleaders, all who work together to go for the gold. You, like the quarterback, call the plays and follow your coach's direction. It still takes practice, though.

You're probably thinking that all the business about dating, sports, college, etc. was a waste of time, since you'll probably be living at a hospital or clinic and won't see the light of day. But you may not need all these team members. Like sands through the hourglass, these are the changing days of your life. The roles of these people will differ depending on your needs.

It's also important to know how to use these professionals in the best way for your diabetes. For example, you may only need to spend a few minutes with the doctor as he or she reviews blood sugar numbers and makes adjustments in your insulin or renews a prescription for you. You might want to spend the rest of the time with your dietitian talking about what to eat to help you get through basketball practice.

So how can you make these visits work to your advantage?

Always take with you the information and data the team needs:
- blood glucose records
- meter with memory
- medications/previous prescriptions
- list of questions
- description of anything unusual that has happened (and the circumstances leading up to it) recorded in your logbook

Bring medical records.
If it's your first visit with a new doctor or team, you're going to want to bring previous medical records. Your parents probably have records of your immunizations, hospitalizations, and previous doctors.

When you see your team members, let them know what's on your mind right away.
Sometimes people wait until the end of the visit to mention their concerns. Whatever is most important to you, get it out there right off the bat!

When you see a new team, tell them what you expect from the start.
You know exactly what you want out of friendships, school, and the sports teams you're on. You also need to have reasonable goals for your health care team. We mentioned some of the services they provide, but you may want to have them do more or

less for you. They don't have crystal balls, so you need to tell them how they can help you. That way, everyone's shooting for the same target.

Sue recently had a young woman tell her that she wasn't quite firm enough in her recommendations. This woman had been trying to lose weight and finally told Sue that she was being "too nice." The woman wanted more confrontation. Sue admits that although she hasn't been paid to get tough before, she's willing to give it a try if it will help!

Be a sponge.

Soak up as much information about diabetes and how to manage it as you can. Jean's doctor once told her, "You have to know your enemy." Now, Jean doesn't think of diabetes as an enemy—she thinks of it more as an inconvenience. But the advice still hits the mark. How can you ward off the effects of diabetes unless you learn as much about it as you can?

Sue diagnosed her own diabetes at the wise old age of 14. At the time, she was trying out a new "grapefruit diet" to lose weight. (One–half grapefruit before each meal and you were guaranteed to lose weight because the acid in the grapefruit supposedly burned fat. Right. If only we were so lucky!) Well, Sue thought the grapefruit was indeed magical because she lost 15 pounds in two weeks. In the meantime, however, she wasn't feeling well. Constant tiredness, rubbery legs, vision changes, and a general "blah" feeling convinced her mother to take her to the doctor. He examined Sue and sent her right back home with a diagnosis of viral flu that she'd just have to fight off herself.

At school, Sue still had difficulty seeing the blackboard; then she got extremely thirsty and started urinating frequently. She learned from some friends that one of the cheerleaders, who had been diagnosed with diabetes two months earlier, had some of the same symptoms. Soon, Sue just knew that she had diabetes. She stopped at the library to read about it and explained everything to her mother while they did the dinner dishes that evening. After listening to Sue's persistent complaints of not feeling well for two days, her mom again called the doctor. This time, Sue brought a urine sample with her. The doctor was skeptical, until Nurse Ratchet brusquely tapped on the door and shook a test tube of bright orange foam at him. Without a word, she closed the door and he looked in disbelief at Sue as he remarked that she had indeed diagnosed her own condition.

So what's the point? Education, even on the most informal level, can lead to better diabetes care.

> **Bottom Line:** You deserve to have the best care and you owe it to yourself to find it!

In Control

CHAPTER 11

GETTING INVOLVED

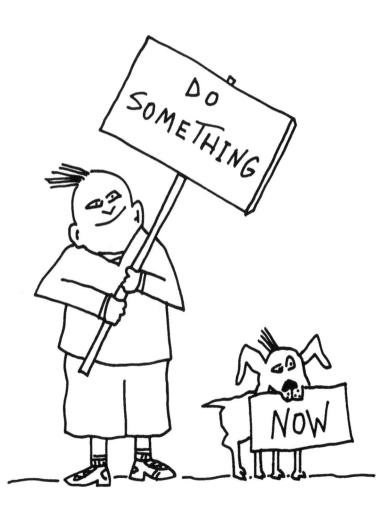

Getting involved with diabetes organizations can be one of the best things you can do for yourself! First of all, making friends with people who have something in common with you (like diabetes, for instance) can help remind you that you aren't alone with the problem. Also, by volunteering for diabetes organizations, we feel like we're helping our diabetes care by practicing what we preach.

What is it that makes this type of experience so valuable? It forces you to be an example for others when you:

- lead a support group.
- have to motivate others to raise money for diabetes research.
- help others take care of themselves.

Some people feel that this may make their life revolve around diabetes too much. Wrong! By focusing on helping others work through diabetes problems, the spotlight comes off you. This makes your diabetes more of a shadow than a focus, something incidental in your life.

Jean and Sue met and developed a friendship because of Type I diabetes. Being leaders in the same organization has helped each achieve personal goals and allowed them to feel they make a difference in the care and education of people with diabetes.

> **Bottom Line:** What goes around, comes around.

CAMP

One of the best things you can do for yourself is to try out a diabetes camp. There are lots of diabetes camps throughout the United States, many of which are sponsored by the American

Diabetes Association. It's a great place to hang out with other people your own age and bond about the horrors and delights of diabetes. Sometimes, seeing what works for someone else is an incentive to try new things.

Diabetes camp can help you make friends, get support from others, and have a blast! (Those who have been to camp before know what we're talking about.) You may even want to volunteer to be a counselor if you like being with kids. Most camps have Counselor–In–Training (CIT) programs that can help you learn the ins and outs of being the perfect camp counselor.

For a complete list of camps or other activities for teens in your area, call your American Diabetes Association Affiliate office or the American Camping Association at (317) 342-8456.

Following is a list of organizations that you can tap into as you live and learn about your diabetes. Some of these places will teach you how to better deal with diabetes, but some of them will offer opportunities to teach others about diabetes. Good luck as you look for the one that's right for you . . . we hope to meet all of you some day at one diabetes event or another!

RESOURCE ORGANIZATIONS & PUBLICATIONS:

American Association of Diabetes Educators
444 North Michigan Ave., Suite 1240
Chicago, IL 60611–3901
1–800–TEAMUP4 (To contact a diabetes educator in your area.)

Resource Organizations and Publications continued.

American Diabetes Association (ADA)
1970 Chain Bridge Road
McLean, VA 22109–0592
1–800–232–3472 (To order publications, cookbooks.)

ADA National Service Center
1660 Duke St.
Alexandria, VA 22314
1–800–232–3472

(For information on local/state affiliates and their activities and programs, including the Youth Leadership Congress and camp.)

Juvenile Diabetes Foundation International
Editorial/World Headquarters
432 Park Ave. S.
New York, NY 10016–8013
1–800–223–1138 (For information on local chapter activities.)

International Diabetic Athletes Association
6829 North 12th St.
Suite 205
Phoenix, AZ 85014
1–602–433–2113

National Diabetes Information Clearinghouse (NDIC)
1 Information Way
Bethesda, MD 20892
1–301–654–3327

Many of the following publications accept articles and they're always looking for interesting personal stories, tips on living with diabetes, and recipe ideas. You could be interviewed or contribute ideas that will help other people with diabetes.

"Diabetes Forecast" (a monthly magazine)
Published by: American Diabetes Association, Inc.
National Service Center
1660 Duke St.
Alexandria, VA 22314
1–800–232–3472 (Subscription Rates: Included with ADA membership at $24/year—$18 is designated for this publication)

"Diabetes Interview" (a monthly newspaper)
Published by: Kings Publishing
3715 Balboa St.
San Francisco, CA 94121
415–387–4002 (Subscription Rates: $14/year, $24/two years)

"Diabetes Self–Management" (a bimonthly magazine)
Published by: R.A. Rapaport Publishing Inc.
150 West 22nd St.
New York, NY 10011
1–800–234–0923 (Subscription Rates: $21/year)

"Countdown" (a quarterly magazine on diabetes research)
Published by: Juvenile Diabetes Foundation International
432 Park Ave. S.
New York, NY 10016
1–800–223–1138 (Subscription Rates: $25/year or free subscription with membership to local JDFI chapter)

INDEX